Cookbooks by Suzy Sable

Suzy Sable's Keto Coloring Cookbook/Book One - FAT BOMBS

Suzy Sable's Keto Coloring Cookbook/Book Two - ICE CREAMS

Keep in the loop:

www.suzysable.com
https://www.facebook.com/suzy.sable.940
https://www.instagram.com/authorsuzysable/
https://twitter.com/authorsuzysable
https://www.pinterest.com/authorsuzysable/

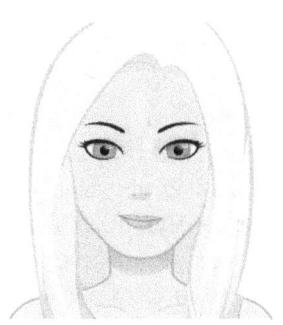

Coloring Pages Preview:

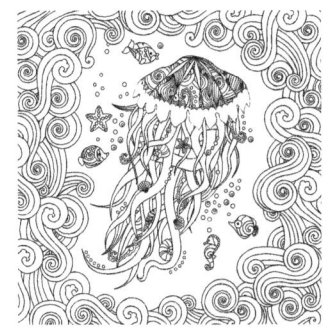
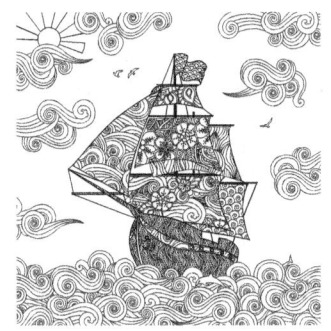
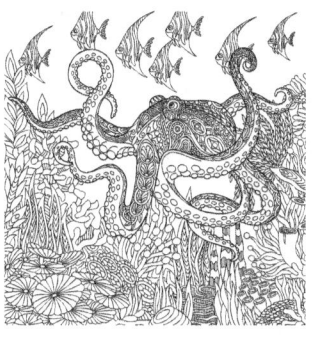
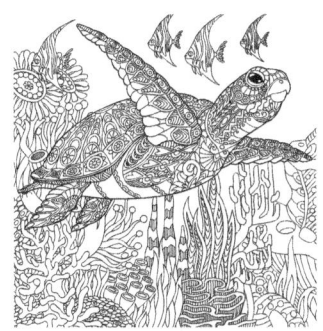
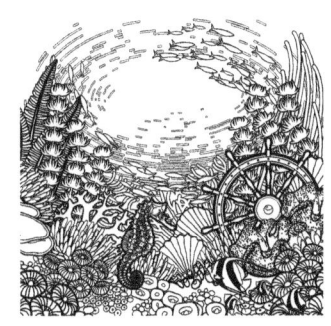
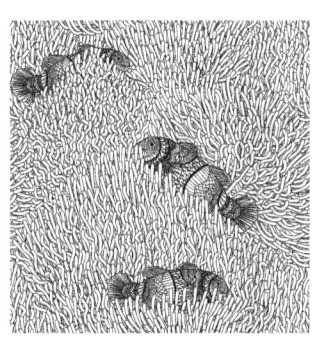
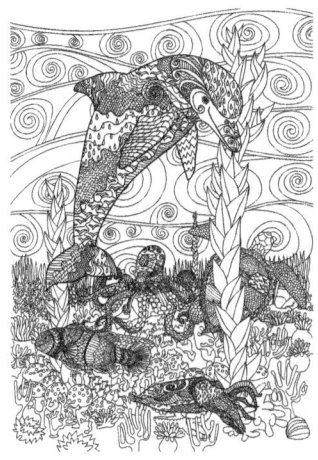
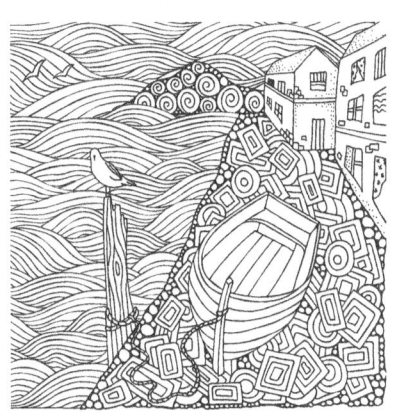
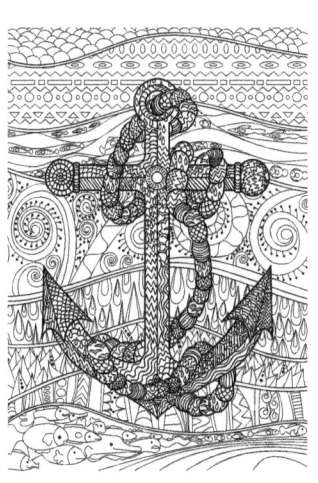
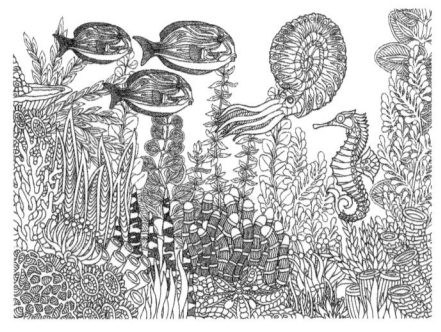

Dedicated to:

Everyone who has ever struggled with weight,
struggled with carbs, sweets, and sugar,
struggled with health.

Making changes is never easy.

Suzy Sable's

KETO

Coloring Cookbook

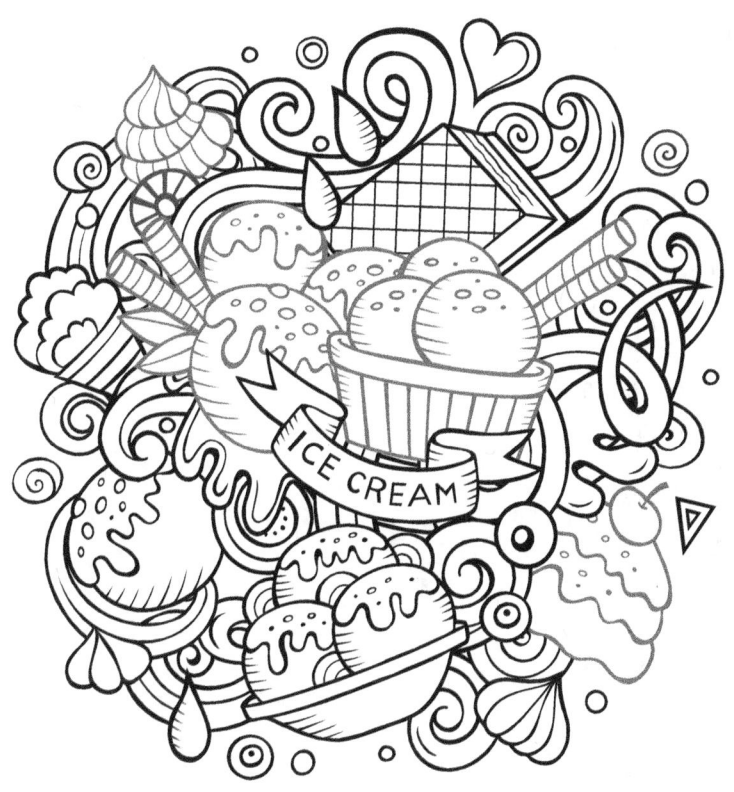

Book Two - ICE CREAMS

Contents: Page:

Keto Basic - 101	11-15
Keto Health & Hygiene Tips	17-19
Keto Products	21-24
Keto Lifestyle Tips	25-30

Artwork & Recipes:

Vanilla	32
Jellyfish	33
Chocolate	36
Sailboat	37
Strawberry	40
Octopus	41
Cookie Dough Bits	43
Cookie Dough	44
Turtle	45
Moose Track Bits	47
Moose Tracks	48
Seahorse	49
Chocolate Chip Mint	52
Clown Fish	53
Graham Cracker Bits	55
Banana Cream Pie	56
Dolphin	57
Keto Brown Sugar	59
Butter Pecan	60
Rowboat	61
Caramel Pecan	64
Anchor	65
Cherry Nut	68
Nautilus	69
*Recipe Notes	72
*Ice Cream Base & Conversion Amounts	73

A Note From The Author:

Thank you so much for buying my book!

My keto journey continues below, but as told in the first book, I started on the ketogenic path as a desperate, 40-pound overweight admitted "Carbo-Girl". I was so consumed by that title, I should've been wearing a Superhero cape. The word "consumed" is apt as well, because carbs were mostly what I ate.

As I debated my weight-loss options, I exceeded 20-pounds overweight, 25-pounds, 30-pounds...hitting an all-time high of 40 pounds overweight! I felt powerless and miserable despite the available wealth of information regarding weight loss, and despite actually *knowing what to do*...less food, more exercise. *Right, right, I got it!* But, I felt stuck. All that information and advice floating around should be empowering, yet I was lost in translation.

Then I planned to attend a large family gathering. Now, these are the times when I'm more acutely aware of my body, because I'm more self-conscious about the weight I've gained since people last saw me.

It'd been easy to be in denial day-to-day, because the weight crept on over a period of months as I just swapped in increasingly floppy clothes, you know, for comfort. (Read: to conceal the weight gain.) But, as I tried on my now ill-fitting, tight outfits for the family get-together, I had to face the music. Staring in the full-length mirror, I dreaded seeing everyone...or rather, I dreaded everyone seeing me.

It's kind of a horrible moment for a person, a depressing kick in the gut. There shouldn't be shame with this kind of struggle, but society is harsh on dysfunction of any kind. And obesity can't be disguised, or hidden, nor is it ever overlooked. Now, I should go into the uplifting rant about ignoring the judgments of society, about everyone having struggles, about loving myself at any weight...but, it had nothing to do with any of that. *I simply didn't want to be this weight anymore!*

So, I was at the family gathering in my schlumpy clothes...My sister and I were watching TV, but in the background, I was tuned in to my brother, *my very fit older brother,* visiting with my dad in the kitchen. And he was talking about the difference in carbs, the whole good-carbs/bad-carbs thing.

I'd heard it before, but for some reason, this time it clicked, the information was finally translating! I suppose it's like they say, you have to hear or see something a number of times before you buy it. Well, I was buying! My brother had become very fit, and it was hard to argue with the visible proof of low-carb eating, especially as I slumped uncomfortably on the couch, under a blanket, in June, hiding my stomach.

However, as I listened...with my Carbo-Girl ears...I felt a little defeated. I didn't think I'd be able to cut carbs to the degree he was talking. In fact, a nutritionist had previously suggested this very thing to me, and I'd commented that so few carbs sounded dangerous. I'd pretty much accused her of being irresponsible. (Yeah, I did that. I probably owe her a fat bomb basket.)

But getting back to the story, when I got home from the trip, desperation set in...or maybe it was motivation...it was one of those "tion"s. With my brother's words ringing in my ears, I researched low-carb and keto eating, as I'm sure you have. And I'm sure you found what I did; when your body doesn't have carbs to burn as energy, it uses *fat!* That really clicked, because I had plenty of fat by then.

I was getting a bit excited about my keto prospects, and I felt the spark of a transforma-tion in the making. It felt like the right time and place for me. Incidentally, I believe transformations need to happen in that way, so let's cut each other a little slack, and give one another the space to progress.

Anyway, I took the keto plunge. Actually, let's be real, my odyssey from Carbo-Girl to Keto-Girl didn't start with a plunge, but more of a tippy-toes first and wade-slowly-in.

So, I dipped in my toes. I got a few keto cookbooks and keto products, thinking *maybe if I keep handy a bunch of keto crap to eat, I can stay on it long enough to kick-start my weight loss.* Suffice it to say, I didn't begin by thinking I'd be able to sustain a keto-eating lifestyle. *No way!*

So, I focused on keto cookbooks offering a lot of desserts and snacks. However, most of the recipes were just, well...*yuck!* And I thought, *I can do better than this!* I've watched my Mom pinch and dash recipes all of my life, and I've always tweaked recipes to fit my tastes...just like my Mom!
(*Hi again, Mom! Your cooking and baking really inspired these books.*)

I have decades of experience in the kitchen as a home cook, so, I got to work because I really wanted to succeed, and I couldn't see sticking with keto unless I could satisfy my sweet-tooth. Because I believe, it's my absolute right as a human being to have dessert every day...maybe with every meal! (Let's be honest, some days it's dessert between meals, before meals.)

So I began experimenting with the unfamiliar keto ingredients, like erythritol and xanthan gum, coconut cream and coconut flour. Not all of my creations were successful, believe me; they can't all be winners! But soon, I had enough palatable staples to stay on keto. And honestly, the intrigue of trying these new recipes kept me engaged and interested in keto life. It wasn't a diet any more; it was an exploration. As the weeks passed, I got excited about my creations and I saw that I was truly losing weight while eating all my new goodies.

So, this series of cookbooks represents a good amount of time and work in my "test kitchen", developing recipes, while staying strictly within keto nutrition guidelines. And along the way, I completely surprised myself! I've kept to the ketogenic diet because *I like it!* I never feel deprived with these yummy recipes, and sometimes I actually feel naughty, as if I've eaten nothing but junk all day!

Another bonus? *I feel good!* My physical health is better, and inflammation that was plaguing my hands and wrists for 5 years is non-existent. My mind is clearer, my energy is higher, and my overall mood and outlook is cheerier and more optimistic. *And, oh yeah...I've lost the 40 pounds!* So, I think I'll stay...

My Keto Coloring Cookbook series is a labor of love, for myself, for my overweight friends and family, and for everyone who's struggling with weight and doesn't know where to turn. If you don't think you can maintain a keto diet, take it from the former Carbo-Girl...*you got this!*

These dessert and snack books will address a variety of goals: non-keto eaters who want to cut carbs significantly, those who want to dip their toes in and experiment with keto eating, or those that intend to go full-on keto. Use these books no matter the route you're taking to weight loss or better health.

Inside these books, I've endeavored to set the reader up for success with tips and recommendations along with easy, delicious recipes to have on hand at all times. These books also contain illustrations, each of which I've selected for its stress-reducing effect.

So, enjoy the books. And if you'd like to be apprised of upcoming books and events, go to my website and sign up for my newsletter, *C-Notes* (Coloring Cookbook Notes) at: **www.suzysable.com.**

Thank you again for buying my book! I wish you every success!

Suzy Sable

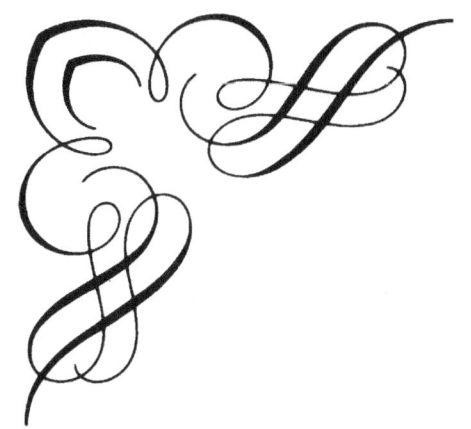
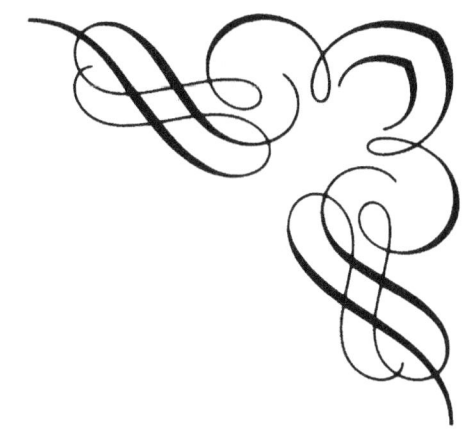

Keto Basic – 101

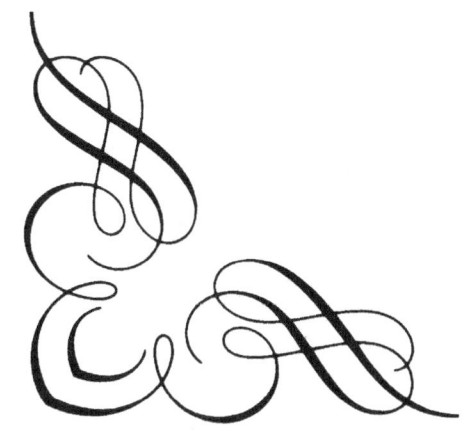
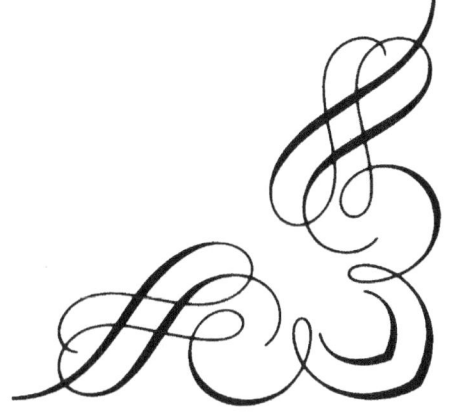

Okay, here's the skinny:

The keto diet boils down to an ultra-low-carb diet that forces your body to change the source of fuel it uses for energy. Instead of chugging away on carbohydrates, your body must tap into stored body fat, which is the process of ketosis.

In a nutshell, your body's first source of energy, glucose, is not available so it goes to the backup source, fat.

The macros necessary to achieve ketosis vary from person to person, but in general, 5 percent of your daily calories will come from carbs (20-50g per day), 20 percent from protein, and 75 percent from fat. The idea here is to find the levels that keep you in ketosis.

How do you know if you're in ketosis? There are methods of testing, urine strips and home blood tests (finger prick). You may also be able to tell by telltale body odor, breath, etc... Now, it's easy to go *ewww* at the mention of these side effects. But hang in there. There are effective fixes for these things, and I'll clue you in to some fixes that worked like a charm for me in the Keto Health & Hygiene section. (So, no, you won't stink.)

I encourage you to be informed about all aspects of the keto diet. And you are on trend here; keto dieting is blowing up right now so there is no shortage of information. I also encourage you to get support, tips, and reputable medical information.

But, to get you started, here's a general list of the Do and Don't foods:

Do's

Meats & Seafood:

Beef, Venison, Lamb, All Pork-chops, roast, bacon, etc., All Poultry-Chicken, Duck, Goose, Quail, etc., All Seafood-Crab, Fish, Shrimp, Scallops, Lobster, Mussels, Octopus, etc.

Dairy:

Butter, Cottage cheese, Cream Cheese, Ricotta Cheese, Queso Blanco, Eggs, Greek Yogurt (Full Fat), Heavy Whipping Cream, Unsweetened Coconut Milk, Unsweetened Almond Milk, Full Fat Creamy Salad Dressings, Full Fat Cheeses, Mozzarella Pearls, etc.

Nuts & Seeds:

Almonds, Macadamia Nuts, Walnuts Flaxseed, Chia Seeds, Hazelnuts, Pine Nuts, Pecans, Brazil Nuts, Walnuts, Sesame Seeds, Pumpkin Seeds

Fruits and Veggies:

Broccoli, Asparagus, Avocados, Bell Peppers, Cabbage, Cauliflower, Herbs, Celery, Alfalfa Sprouts, Lettuce, Zucchini, Cucumbers, Mushrooms, Pickles, Radishes, Salad Greens, Scallions, and for fruit...Berries

Don't's

Meats & Seafood:

Most Deli Meat, Hot Dogs, Tofu, Sausage and other meats with fillers

Dairy:

Milk, Sweetened Almond Milk, Sweetened Coconut Milk, Regular Soy Milk, Regular Yogurt

Nuts & Seeds:

Cashews, Chestnuts, Pistachios. Peanuts should also be avoided, but can be eaten in moderation.

Fruits and Veggies:

Apples, Apricots, Bananas, Cherries, Boysenberries, Dates, Plums, Raisins, Prunes, Kiwi, Honeydew Melon, Cantaloupe, Mangos, Oranges, Peaches, Mangos, Grapes, Pineapples, Potatoes, Sweet Potatoes, Yams, Winter Squash, Water Chestnuts, Turnips, Beans, Artichokes, Chickpeas, Corn, Leeks, Eggplant, Parsnips, Peas

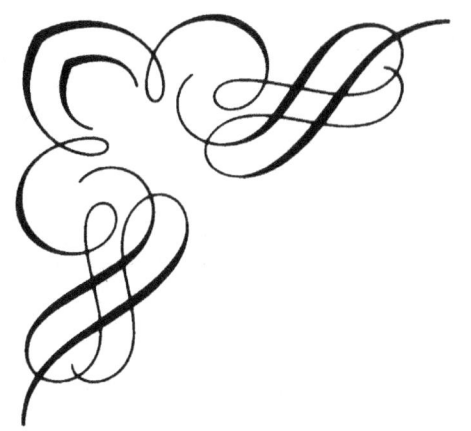
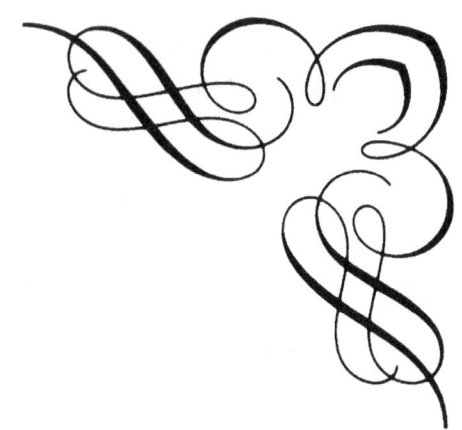

Keto Health & Hygiene Tips

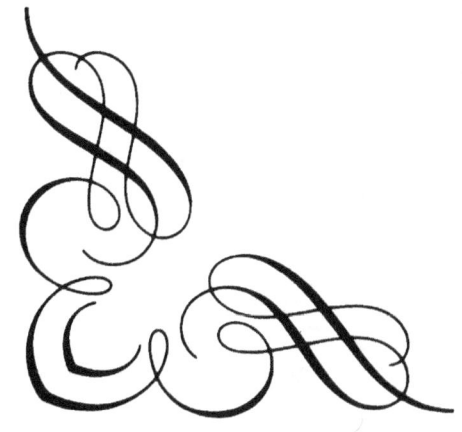
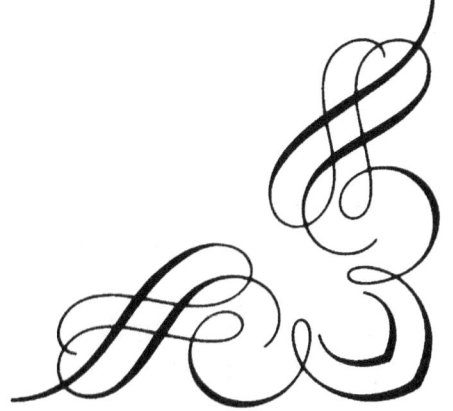

I'm not going to lie, there are some humbling side effects to keto eating. This section addresses the most common, so here we go...

Keto Body Odor

Yes, you can start to smell a little funky. If you want to know the reasons for this, go for it. Look it up. But, I'm more interested in the solution. I've found that what does the trick for me is to spray some Apple Cider Vinegar under my arms and pat it in. I let the ACV dry and apply my deodorant as usual. This lasts me all day, but you can always carry a small spray bottle and spritz if necessary.

The apple cider vinegar will smell astringent at first, but once it dries, it's a non-issue. If the astringency bothers you, or you simply want to add scent, add essential oils to the vinegar. Most essential oils don't mix well with the vinegar, but I really like adding equal drops of pink grapefruit and sweet orange to the ACV. Experiment and find your preference.

Keto Flu

Electrolytes, electrolytes, ELECTROLYTES! I drink 8 Oz. of Powerade Zero or Gatorade Zero a day. (Make sure to get Zero-the sugar free drink.) Also drink plenty of water, get enough sleep, and don't over-exercise. There is a wealth of information regarding keto flu. I do recommend you join an online community or subscribe to a reputable keto newsletter for tips and support.

Keto Teeth

So, this is purely anecdotal, but I was on keto for some time and while flossing, I felt a big chunk come loose. In the sink, it looked like a piece of almond I'd been eating...or at least I prayed it was because it felt more like part of the coating of my tooth had come off!

Researching it to see if I needed to stop keto and see a dentist *tout de suite*, I read an almost identical recount of the experience...and the woman recounting her story had gone to the dentist and been told it was *plaque...falling right off!* I was delighted, because my hygienist had always commented on the amount of plaque I had...*bing! Carbo-Girl teeth!* Shortly thereafter, I went to the dentist to make sure all was well, and this was confirmed. I got a gold star for plaque reduction.

However, good-news/bad-news sitch. I also started to get a creeping-up-from-the-gums browning...so called "keto spots". The dark spots are reportedly caused by a different bacteria from the change of diet. My solution to that is to gargle with Colgate Optic White. Now, I'm going to warn you, it's unpleasant-tasting, and it can burn. (I'm really selling it, huh?) But it works. Try a mouthwash with peroxide or baking soda to address the darkening.

In addition, I switched to a battery-operated toothbrush. I definitely yield to dental advice, though, and recommend you see your dentist about any oral concerns, and be sure to tell them about your change in diet.

Keto Constipation

Be ready for an over-share: I've always pooped like a champion. But when I started keto, I hit a bit of a feces slump. Happily, this was easy to overcome. Here's the combo that did it for me:

*8 Oz of electrolyte drink per day (Zero carb, like Powerade Zero or Gatorade Zero.)

*1 Serving of MCT Oil per day. (I recommend Perfect Keto: See *Keto Products* section.)

*1 1000mg Lysine pill per day. I chew it, though a bit yucky, to get the most benefit. (Also great for eliminating cold sores. Chew one a day, or the moment you feel that telltale cold sore tingle on your lip. And don't use moistening agents on a cold sore, even if they proclaim to be a "cure". Cold sores flourish in moisture. But, I digress. Back to keto constipation...)

*Add Fiber. I find an easy way to do this is to add ground flax seed to sauces, or ground meats. Add just a bit and it won't alter the flavor, but it will get your back on track...or back on the toilet. (Too much? Sorry.)

When I add each of these every day, I'm back to system regularity.

Multi-Vitamin

I recommend taking a multi-vitamin supplement for the changes from your keto diet. Consult a professional regarding which supplementation you require, making mention of the fact that you're on a keto diet that restricts certain nutrients. Your healthcare administrator can help you choose one that addresses these changes.

*Consult your health care professional with changes to diet and supplements.

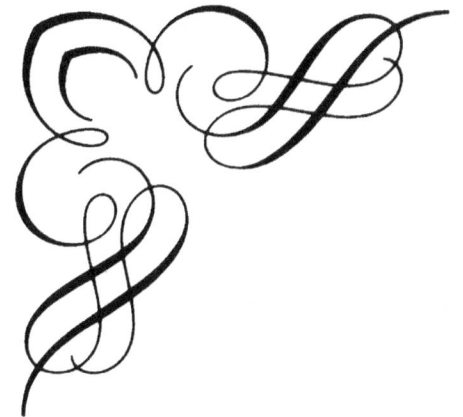
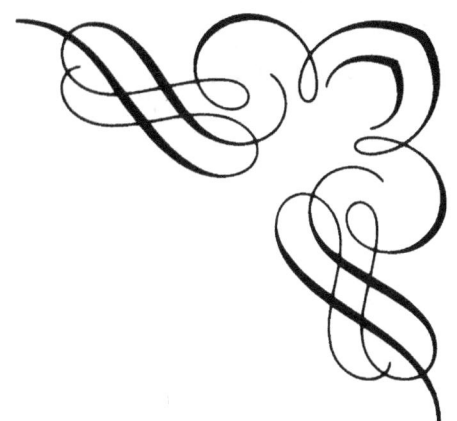

Keto Products

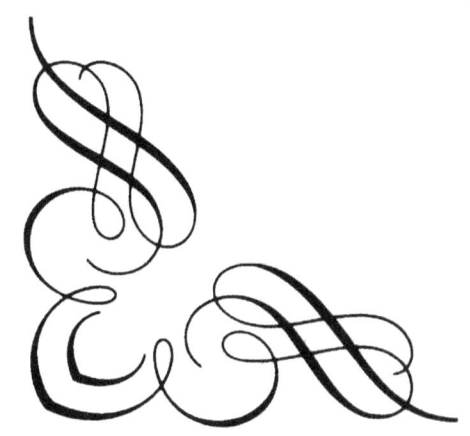
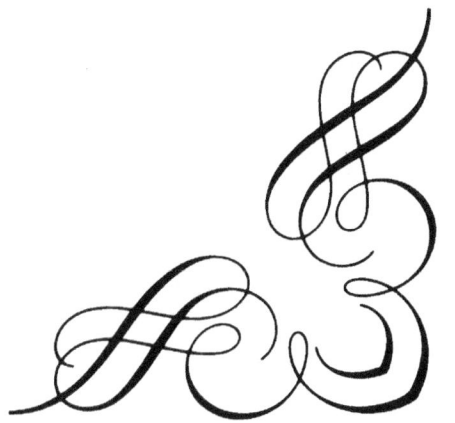

It's a wonderful time for Keto-ers. The ketogenic lifestyle is gaining understanding and popularity, so there are tons of products, recommendations, blogs, websites, groups, organizations, and no end of information. Here, I'll simply recommend a few of my favorite products and the reason why...

Ice Cream Maker

I'm recommending this ice cream maker I found on Amazon because it's a workhorse for the price. I've made at least a hundred batches and mini-batches of ice cream with this model while perfecting the recipes for this book. This ice cream maker is extremely easy to use, and easy to clean. The bucket is a turquoise color. Here's the description:

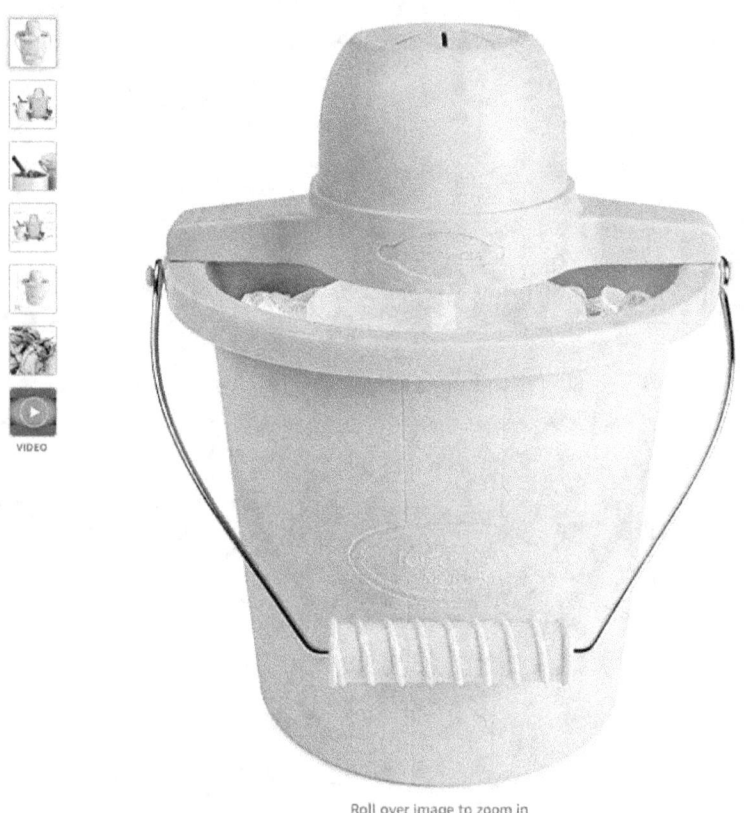

VIDEO

Roll over image to zoom in

Nostalgia ICMP400BLUE 4-Quart Electric Ice Cream Maker with Easy Carry Handle
by Nostalgia

☆ ☆ ☆ ☆ ☆ ∨   970 customer reviews | 125 answered questions

Amazon's Choice for "ice cream machine"

Price: **$28.76** ✓prime

Pay $28.76 $19.80 after using available Amazon Rewards Visa Card Points.

Free Amazon tech support included ∨

Style Name: **Ice Cream Maker**

Bundle Set	Ice Cream Maker
- -	$28.76 ✓prime

- 4-QUART CAPACITY - Great for party time or snack time, this unit makes 4-quarts of delicious ice cream, frozen yogurt or gelato - enough to feed everyone!
- NOSTALGIA ICE CREAM KITS - Unit works perfectly with all Nostalgia ice cream kits - try the Vanilla Crème, Chocolate or Strawberry Ice Cream Mixes (ICP825VAN8PK, ICP825CHOC8PK, ICP825STRAW8PK), or the Premium Ice Cream Starter Kit (ISK3).
- CLEANUP IS EASY - With a plastic bucket that wipes away messes with ease, cleaning up afterwards is a breeze.
- SEE-THRU LID - To store leftover ice cream in the freezer, a see-thru lid is included that fits on top of the canister.
- EASY-CARRY HANDLE - A carrying handle attached to the bucket makes it convenient to move your ice cream wherever it needs to go.
- NO MANUAL EFFORT NEEDED - A powerful electric motor does all the churning, so no intensive stirring or manual effort is required!
- MOTOR LOCK - The electric motor locks into place, keeping all parts secure.
- RECIPES - Use your own recipes, or follow the recipes included in the manual to get started making delicious and creamy ice cream.

Silicone Measuring Cups

No, I don't work for Amazon, nor do I receive any commission for sales ☺. But, I did find these perfect measuring cups there. The reason I'm recommending them is that in addition to being good measuring cups, they're great for melting butter, coconut oil, or anything else needed. I've been able to heat things to boiling and grip these containers without an oven mitt. They're dishwasher safe, microwave safe, and BPA free.

I recommended these in Book One - FAT BOMBS as well, since they're a one-container fat-bomb-maker for those recipes. Here's the description:

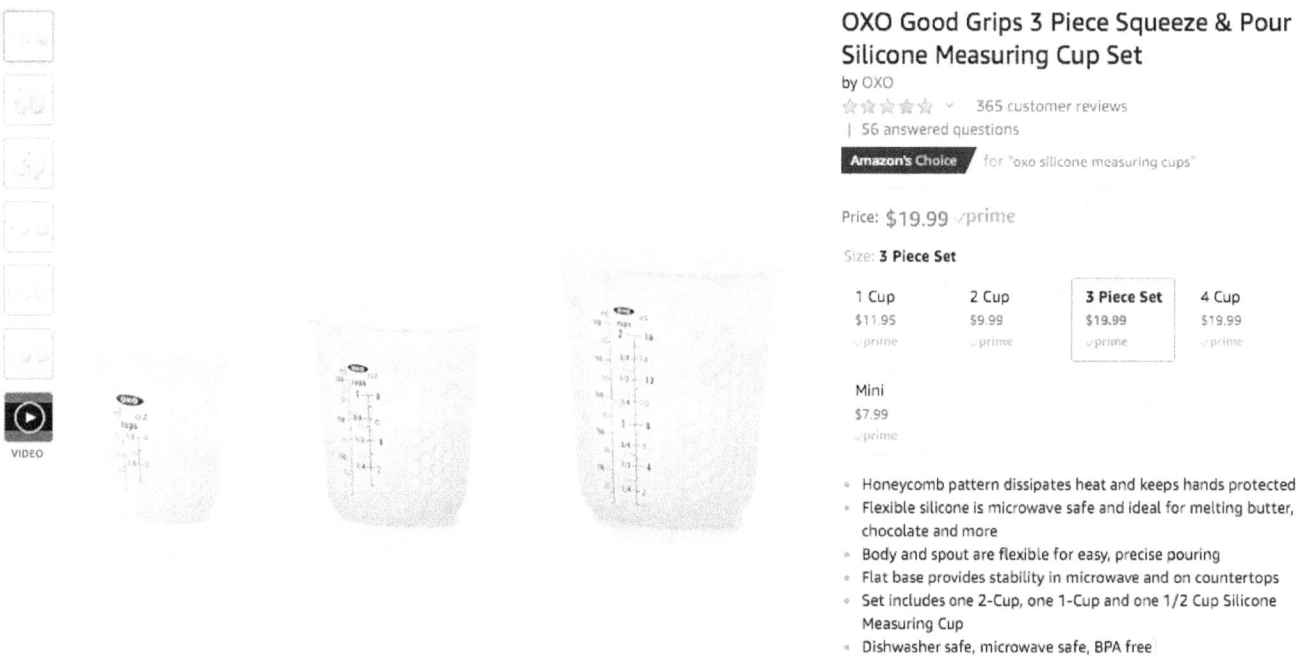

OXO Good Grips 3 Piece Squeeze & Pour Silicone Measuring Cup Set
by OXO
☆☆☆☆☆ ⌄   365 customer reviews
| 56 answered questions

Amazon's Choice for "oxo silicone measuring cups"

Price: $19.99 ✓prime

Size: **3 Piece Set**

1 Cup	2 Cup	**3 Piece Set**	4 Cup
$11.95	$9.99	$19.99	$19.99
✓prime	✓prime	✓prime	✓prime

Mini
$7.99
✓prime

- Honeycomb pattern dissipates heat and keeps hands protected
- Flexible silicone is microwave safe and ideal for melting butter, chocolate and more
- Body and spout are flexible for easy, precise pouring
- Flat base provides stability in microwave and on countertops
- Set includes one 2-Cup, one 1-Cup and one 1/2 Cup Silicone Measuring Cup
- Dishwasher safe, microwave safe, BPA free

Food and Drink Recommendations

For sugar free syrups, all the syrups I used, except for banana are Torani brand. You can find the flavored syrups used in this cookbook on (yes, you guessed it) Amazon, but you can also go straight to the Torani company website. There, they offer a larger selection of sugar free syrups. Make sure you're ordering their *Sugar Free* syrups, though. They didn't have a sugar free banana as of the publishing date of this book, so I used Da Vinci for my banana cream pie ice cream.

As for MCT Oil, I recommend Perfect Keto Products especially their MCT Oil Powder-Unflavored. Mostly I love this because I don't drink coffee. I tend to drink water, and I was hesitant to put something called *oil* in my water. I thought it would taste oily-greasy, but Perfect Keto doesn't. It doesn't really taste like anything at all, nor does it have any after-taste.

It tastes pretty much like water and helps me stay in keto by providing some of the fat I need in addition to getting me quickly back in ketosis if I go off. The Perfect Keto brand has a great selection of flavors and functions, such as MCT oils, collagen powders, protein powders, etc.

If you want the unflavored MCT Oil, it can be tricky because several canisters look alike. Read carefully, looking just below the square logo for the flavor.

Perfect Keto MCT Oil Powder   Isopure Banana Cream Protein Powder

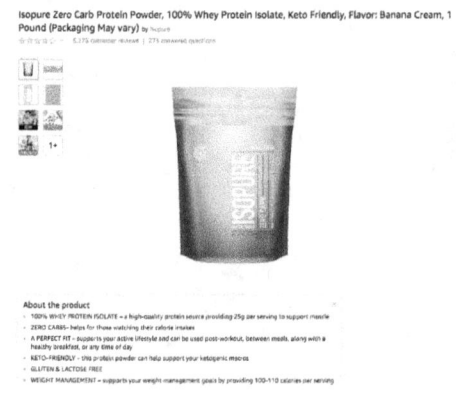

For protein powder, I recommend the above Isopure Banana Cream Protein Powder-because it's truly yummy! Great taste and low carbs, what's not to like? But if you're not partial to banana cream, choose a protein powder carefully. Most are *loaded* with carbs.

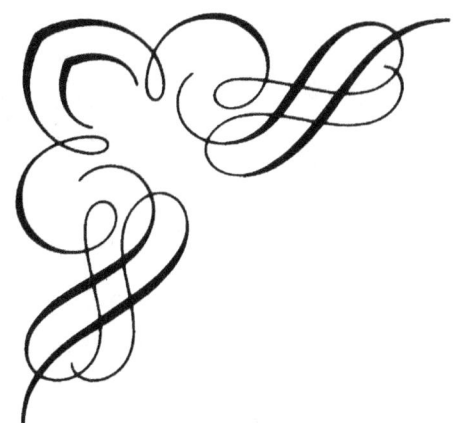
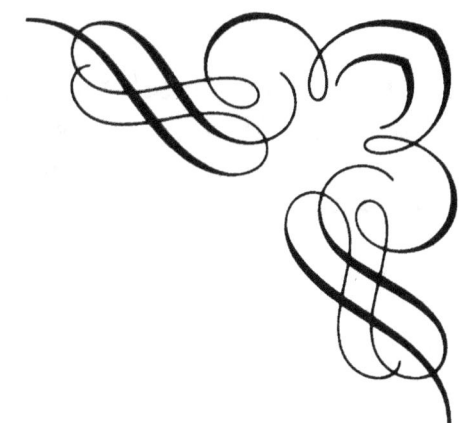

Keto Lifestyle Tips

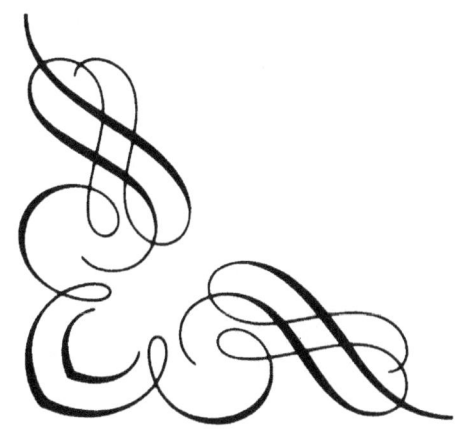
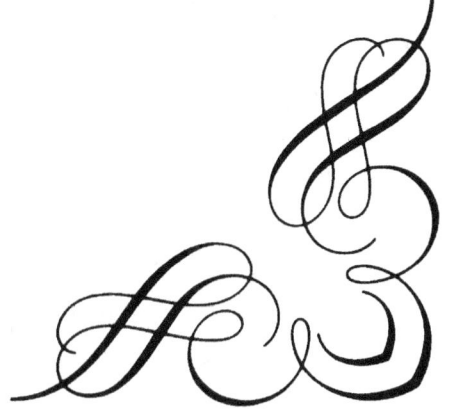

A Preface

Before I launch into my suggestions and tips, I'd like to give you a hint of my personality, so you get a sense of where I'm coming from. That way, if it meshes with your personality, you can use these tips and if not, you can take things with a grain of salt, or discard them altogether and forge your unique path.

So...I don't like to be told *No.* If I set my mind to something, I'm going to find a way to make it happen. And if I'm not buying what you're selling, you're probably not going to change my mind. In that vein, I also don't like to feel deprived. If I'm told I can't have something, the rebellious side of me wants it all the more.

Don't get me wrong, I'm not easily manipulated or reversed-psychology-ed (not a word, ☺) so if I don't want something, I won't want it just because someone tells me I can't have it. No, I know my own mind. I'm saying, if I want something and I'm told I can't have it, like a dessert...well, my brain short-circuits. I go into a thought-loop about that dessert and I don't emerge from the vortex until the morsel is in my mouth.

So I've figured, *for myself, for my personality,* if there's some treat I want, I'd better find a way to make that happen within the keto parameters, because it's happening one way or the other!

Now there are two schools of thought for keto eating; clean vs. dirty. Both are paths to a keto lifestyle, neither better than the other, as long as it works for you. As you've probably guessed, my path is to go a little dirty. I find this way is more convenient and cheaper, making it more practical for me. And if I'm being honest, it also suits my personality...it sounds more fun and permissive.

So, with that in mind, I'll propose my strategies.

Every Day

The only way I've been able to stay on keto is to have a plethora of handy foods available. In fact, the times I've slipped, I've hardly had any choices available. And it's not that the couple of things I had weren't perfectly yummy; it's just a psychological glitch with me that if I only have one thing to eat *I don't want that.* This doesn't apply to people. I can be happy and satisfied with my one person, but when it comes to one food...no! Give me variety!

So, I spend little spurts of time in the kitchen each week. My strategy has been to make a bunch of things, fat bombs, Ice creams, meats, blanched broccoli, and cut celery stalks. (Yes, when I eat celery I serve myself whole, de-leafed stalks in a pretty jar or wide vase because the little chopped-in-half celery sticks seem stingy and sad. Same with lettuce. I like the long lettuce heart leaves in a pretty vase.)

I'll also crockpot a whole bag of chicken, and bake 2-3 pounds of ground turkey or ground beef in a cake pan (with a couple tablespoons of ground flaxseed to replace bread or crumbs for bulk and fiber). Once baked, I cut the meat into American Cheese-size squares, to be topped with the cheese when reheated.

And then I'm set. With different cheeses, flavorings, seasonings, toppings, not to mention easy cheese snacks and nuts...I have a week's worth of grab-able food.

Social Gatherings

There are plenty of tips out there, and I won't rehash how you should stay away from this and that at social gatherings. There are many ways you can approach social gatherings, vacations, and holidays. There are as many creative strategies as there are people. Do what works for you, but I'll suggest two of mine.

Strategy 1 has to do with carb-cycling. You'll find many mentions of the need to come off keto for periods. I find that when I come off keto, my inflammation acts up and my hands and wrists start to hurt. However, for short periods, it seems to give my plateauing keto metabolism a kick-start. So I plan short keto breaks four to five times a year, corresponding with my favorite celebrations. This is a no-guilt, much needed, healthy break. At these times, I even eat *gasp* bad carbs, without a blink!

I'm not trying to sabotage you here. So, if you've never gained a pound, staying strictly on your diet regimen during all holidays, then keep a strict keto regimen. That suits you. This book has plenty of ice creams to deck the halls, (and in my upcoming books keto holidays, breads, cakes, cookies, cheesecakes, crackers, chips, and fudge), so you can maintain ketosis rather than gorging on high-carb cookies, candy, bakery, and sugar-loaded fudge.

However, if you've been apt to fa-la-la 'cuz tis the season, plan your 3-4 keto breaks on your year-round calendar to coincide with your favorite holidays. But, don't go overboard. No taking a keto break because it's National Anthem Day (March 3rd).

After the break, get back to keto...if you'd like. With the decadent foods I've developed, I've become so comfortable with keto eating, that I don't worry I won't get back to it. As another incentive to return to tasty keto eating, I don't feel very good when I'm off it. As I mentioned, my hands and wrists hurt almost unbearably, but that's not all. Off of keto I have stomach troubles, my mood tanks, along with my energy...and my high-carb brain fog returns. So, for me, I don't sweat the bad carb blips; I enjoy them tremendously albeit briefly. Because I know I'll return to keto to feel good.

Strategy 2 is for when I'm at a celebration or holiday, but I'm eating keto. When I think about it, the main dish is usually turkey, ham, beef, goose, duck, etc... Meat! And there's usually a variety of cheeses, and nuts. But I have to forego all the carby breads, bakery, chips, and starchy veggies or potato dishes as well as the sweet and/or alcoholic drinks.

Sooo, if I'm on keto, I make sure I have something just for me. I bring a tasty keto banana cream drink, chocolate drink, or Zero electrolyte drink (fruit punch, mixed berry, grape, etc...) *and* some keto treats, just for me; delicious macadamia nuts, almonds, or some of the gooey fat bombs from my first book, etc... I slip these onto my plate and I have something delicious, just for me.

If I'm staying over at a friend or relative's house, I squirrel away plenty of treats, tucking some in my room, some in a corner of the fridge or freezer. (Or, in winter here in Minnesota, I can store them on a porch, three-season room, or garage.) I've become accustomed to traveling with a variety of keto foods as well as my MCT Oil and electrolyte drinks. This can take a little additional planning, but it's doable for me.

For Valentine's Day, I make fat bombs or ice cream in a heart mold. For other killer candy days, like Halloween, I make them in a ghost mold. You get the idea. And stayed tuned for your birthday. I'll be releasing a cake edition in this series!

For travel/vacations, I use the same strategies. Either I'm off keto, or I bring foods with me.

Also, I suggest here, and in other places in this book, that you venture into some form of keto support or info group online. You want tips, believe me, you'll get tips. People are very creative and ingenious and there's invariably some nugget to be mined from these sites. Moving on...

Restaurants

Fast food is limited, but every one of them has options. It's a matter of ordering the sandwich without ketchup or other sauces, and stripping off the bun. And of course, no fries or potatoes, desserts, shakes, or other sugary drinks. Pretty much just meat, cheese, water, and coffee.

I thought I'd really miss the buns, but startlingly, I find the food much tastier without them. I mean, think about it. These fast food places don't give you inches-thick, juicy meat. You get this shriveled, almost cracker-thin piece of meat with cheese melted almost to death.

So, go for the double or triple cheeseburger or bacon cheeseburger, discard the bun, and bite into a surprising burst of flavor. Same goes for the breakfast sandwiches. Without the English muffin...mmmm...*magnificent!* (Warning, you may look a little strange eating it. My dad commented that what I was doing was weird...☺ But, that was just an added bonus!)

At sit-down restaurants, you'll find a bigger variety, but not so fast... Be mindful of what comes smothered on your order. Think through the sauces, breads, side dishes, etc... But again, make sure to load things up with all the keto goodies, and you won't feel like you're eating like a gen-pop prisoner.

Take advantage. Have your meat or seafood with tons of butter, garlic butter, parsley butter, avocado, cheese, bacon, healthy oils, sour cream, and have sides of cottage cheese, cream cheese, broccoli in butter or cheese sauce, and on and on. You get nuts and cheeses. You get berries. There's really a great variety from which to choose.

For Couples/Partners/Families (however you identify your pack) who aren't all on keto

Most of what you'll eat is what anyone would eat in a meal. After all...keto is food! You'll just want to substitute the carb stuff your family's eating for your keto goodies. For instance, eat the meat, loading it with cheese, bacon, butter, avocado, olive oil or other healthy oil, almonds, walnuts, or any of a great variety of satisfying keto extras.

And don't forget the extra flavors: pickle, onion, garlic, mustard, herbs. Add seasonings instead of sauces, like Cajun, chipotle, Sriracha, Chinese Five Spice, Season-All salt, etc... (Avoid the ketchup, and other bottled sauces-just read the carbs on them! Some boast more carbs than ice cream!)

Then eat a keto vegetable, again loading it with keto goodies, because keto eating is not meant to be flavorless or dissatisfying. *Far from.* Eating a high amount of fat, with so many flavorings, seasonings, and toppings is very satisfying and it provides a steady satiation without the sugar highs and lows. Serve rich Alfredo or cheese sauce over spiralized veggies or riced cauliflower. And *then...*savor one of the ice creams in this book.

You get the idea. Eating with the family can be pretty straightforward, so my main suggestion in this couples/partners/families section is to provide a list of things for your loved-ones to get you at the grocery store.

And, I'm not talking about weekly shopping here. I'm talking about little surprises for him/her/them to get for you. My sig-other expressed frustration that he couldn't get me any of the old, tried-and-true sweets anymore...my favorite candies and caramel corn. And truth be told, I missed receiving his thoughtful treats. But it turned out to be a very easy fix, replace caramel corn with macadamia nuts and bites of candy with mozzarella pearls. It really wasn't about what he got me...it's just that he got me.

Going keto doesn't mean all joy of life has to go. Because it's the little things that bring joy of life and it's easy to make room for that. So, when you're making a lifestyle change, make room for the counted-on comforts, the tried-and-true traditions, and the love.

And so, on to the love...

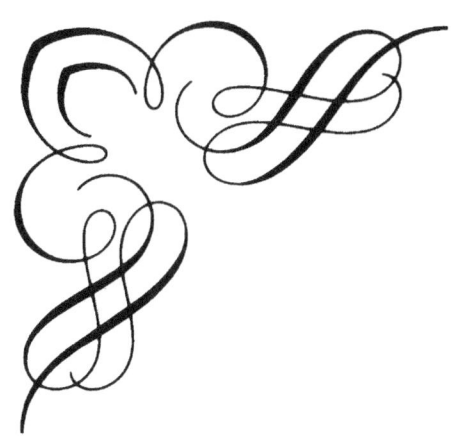
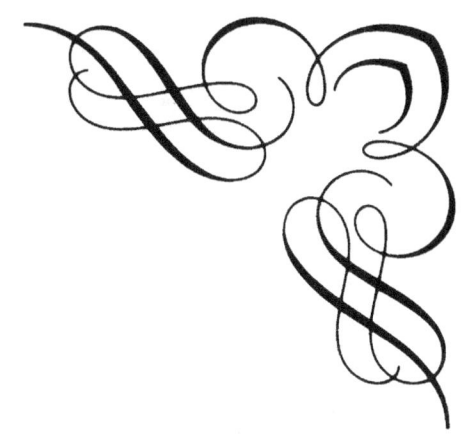

ARTWORK & RECIPES

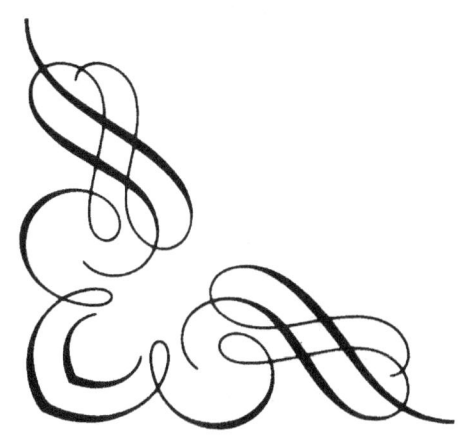
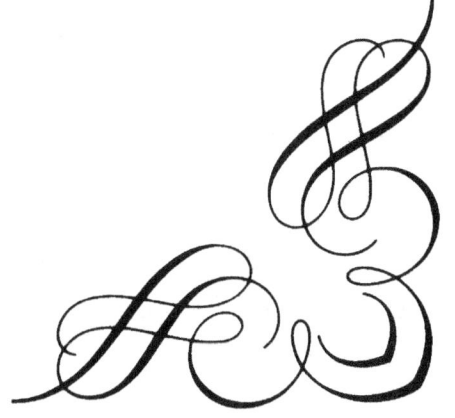

Vanilla
(Makes 2 Quarts = 16 Servings of 1/2 Cup)

2 C	Unsweetened Coconut Milk
2 Cans	Unsweetened Coconut Cream
2 T	Erythritol
1/2 C	Sugar Substitute (Such as Splenda)
1/2 t	Salt
1 1/2 T	Vanilla Extract
1 t	Xanthan Gum
2 t	Sugar Substitute (Such as Stevia or Splenda)
1 C	Sugar Free Vanilla Bean Syrup (Such as Torani)

*You will need rock salt and a good supply of ice.

In a large saucepan, add the first six ingredients. Warm the mixture on medium-low to low heat, dissolving the lumps of coconut cream. This mixture doesn't need to get hot; the idea is to dissolve the lumps. Stir occasionally to see if the lumps are melted, but you don't need to babysit this.

Once the lumps are dissolved, refrigerate the base ingredients until chilled. (Chill your ice cream canister at this time-if recommended in the ice cream maker's instructions.)

In a tiny bowl, mix together the xanthan gum and sugar substitute and set aside until base mixture is chilled. When base mixture is chilled, add the Vanilla Bean syrup and pour into a blender. Sprinkle the xanthan/sugar substitute mixture on top of liquid and blend for 30 seconds to a minute.

Empty the liquid ice cream mixture into your ice cream canister, using a spatula if necessary. Churn, following the ice cream maker's instructions.

Eat immediately as soft serve, or pour into a freezer-safe container, allowing for expansion of ingredients. Chill 2-4 hours.

Nutrition Per Serving (1/2 Cup):
Calories: 102; Fat: 10g: Sat Fat 10g; Protein: 0g; Carbs: 1g as Erythritol

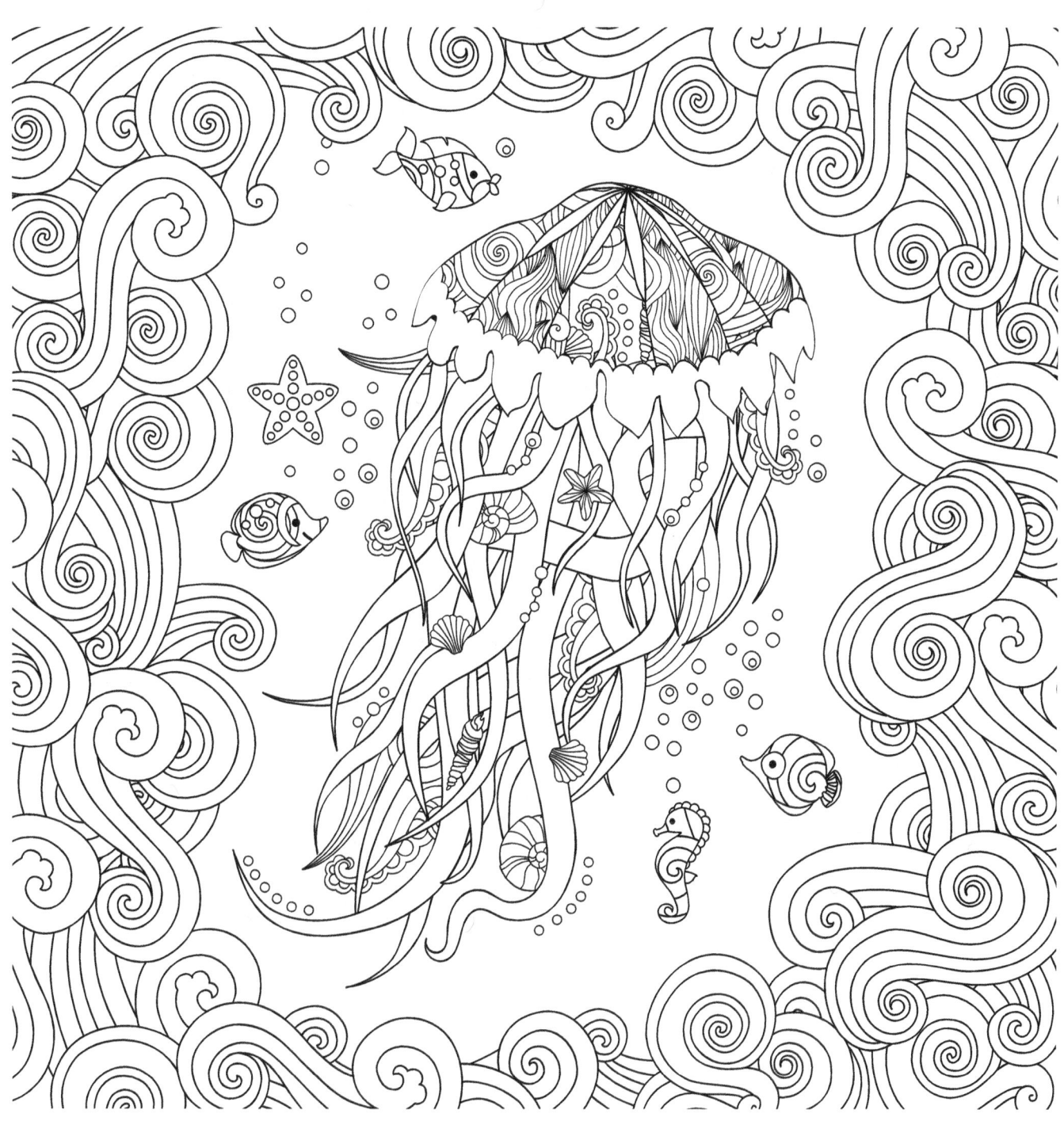

Chocolate
(Makes 2 Quarts = 16 Servings of 1/2 Cup)

2 C	Unsweetened Coconut Milk
2 Cans	Unsweetened Coconut Cream
2 T	Erythritol
1/2 C	Sugar Substitute (Such as Stevia or Splenda)
1/2 t	Salt
1 t	Xanthan Gum
2 t	Sugar Substitute (Such as Splenda)
1 C	Sugar Free Chocolate Syrup (Such as Torani)
1/4 C	Unsweetened Cocoa Powder

*You will need rock salt and a good supply of ice.

In a large saucepan, add the first five ingredients. Warm the mixture on medium-low to low heat, dissolving the lumps of coconut cream. This mixture doesn't need to get hot; just dissolve the lumps. Stir occasionally to see if the lumps are melted, but you don't need to babysit this.

Once the lumps are dissolved, refrigerate the base ingredients until chilled. (Chill your ice cream canister at this time-if recommended in the ice cream maker's instructions.)

In a tiny bowl, mix together the xanthan gum and sugar substitute and set aside until the base mixture is chilled. When the base mixture is chilled, add the chocolate syrup and cocoa powder, and pour into a blender. Sprinkle the xanthan/sugar substitute mixture on top and blend for 30 seconds to a minute.

Empty the liquid ice cream mixture into your ice cream canister, using a spatula if necessary. Churn, following the ice cream maker's instructions.

Eat immediately as soft serve, or pour into a freezer-safe container, allowing for expansion of ingredients, and chill 2-4 hours.

Nutrition Per Serving (1/2 Cup):
Calories: 105; Fat: 10g: Sat Fat 10g; Protein: 0g; Carbs: 1g as Erythritol

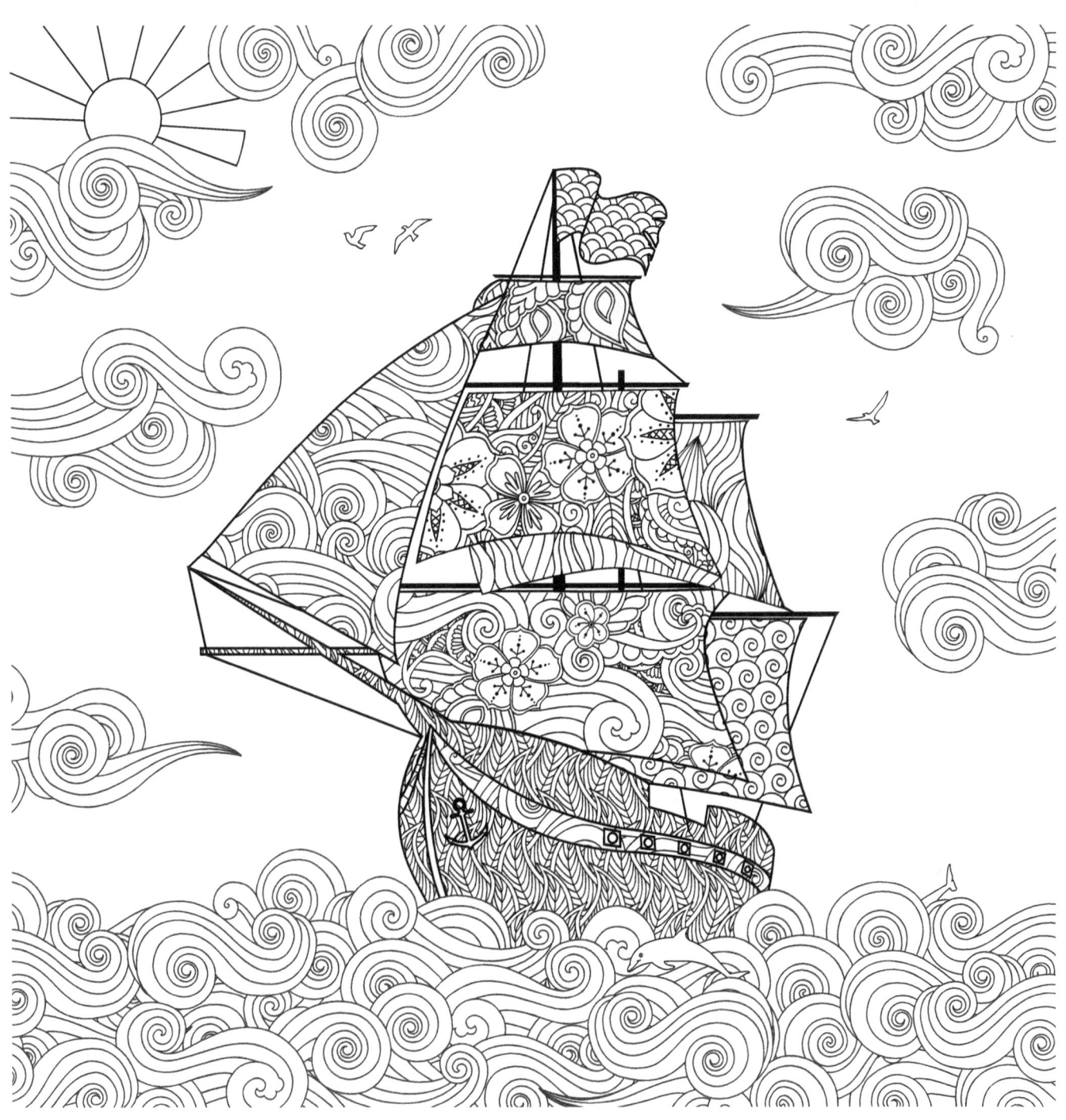

Strawberry
(Makes 2 Quarts = 16 Servings of 1/2 Cup)

2 C	Unsweetened Coconut Milk
2 Cans	Unsweetened Coconut Cream
2 T	Erythritol
1/2 C	Sugar Substitute (Splenda or such)
1/2 t	Salt
1 1/2 T	Vanilla Extract
1 t	Xanthan Gum
2 t	Sugar Substitute (Such as Stevia or Splenda)
1 C	Sugar Free Strawberry Syrup (Such as Torani)

*You will need rock salt and a good supply of ice.

In a large saucepan, add the first six ingredients. Warm the mixture on medium-low to low heat, dissolving the lumps of coconut cream. As always stated, this mixture doesn't need to get hot; just dissolve the lumps, stirring occasionally to see if they're melted.

Once the lumps are dissolved, refrigerate the base ingredients until chilled. (Chill your ice cream canister at this time-if recommended in the ice cream maker's instructions.)

In a tiny bowl or ramekin, mix together the xanthan gum and sugar substitute and set aside until your base mixture is chilled. When the base mixture is chilled, add the strawberry syrup and pour into a blender. Sprinkle the xanthan/sugar substitute mixture on top and blend for 30 seconds to a minute.

Empty the liquid mixture into your ice cream canister, using a spatula if necessary. Churn, following the ice cream maker's instructions.

Eat immediately as soft serve, or pour into a freezer-safe container, allowing for expansion of ingredients, and chill 2-4 hours.

Nutrition Per Serving (1/2 Cup):
Calories: 102; Fat: 10g: Sat Fat 10g; Protein: 0g; Carbs: 1g as Erythritol

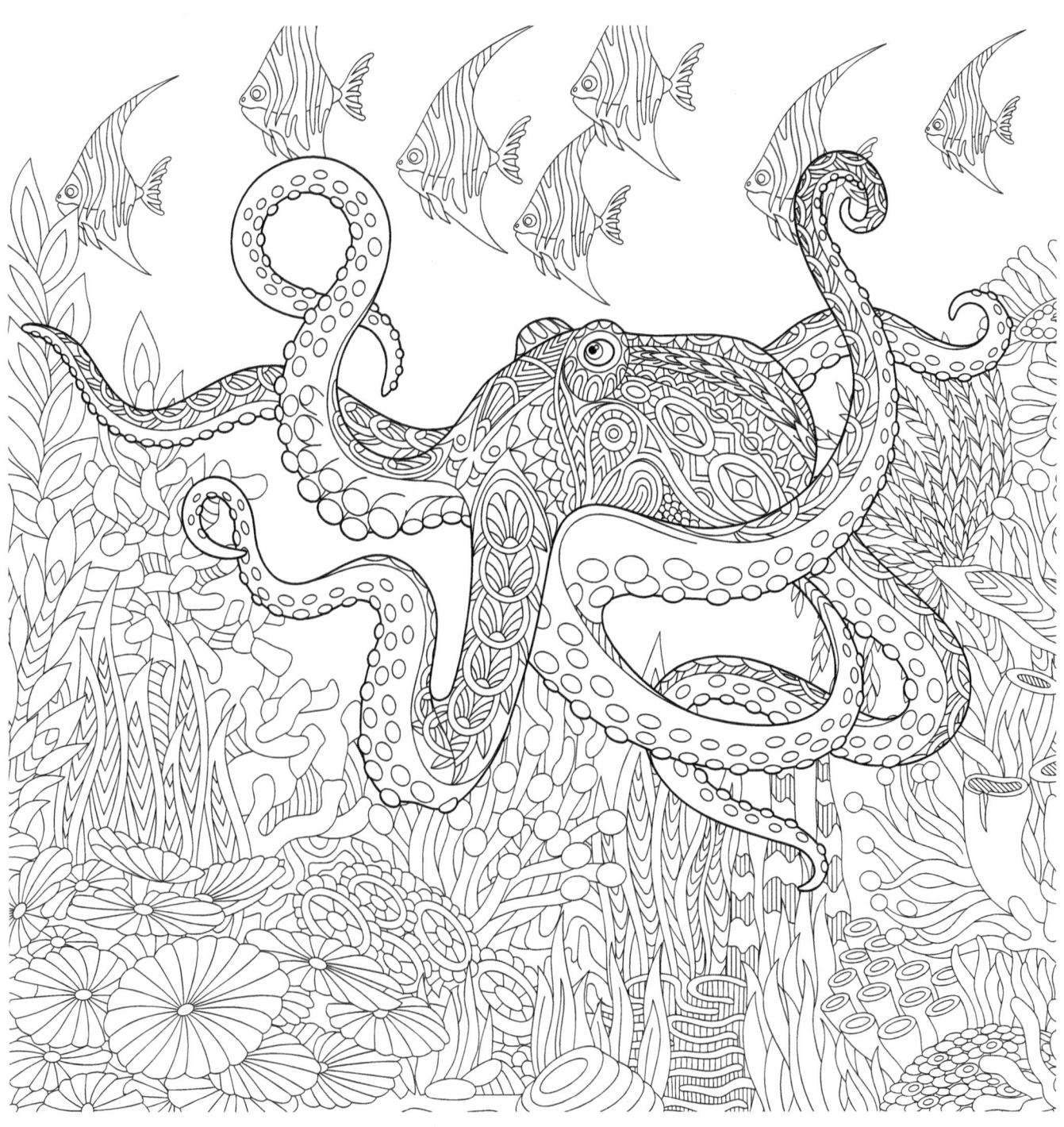

Cookie Dough Bits
This recipe is modified from Book One - Fat Bombs
(This makes enough for the 2 Quart Ice Cream recipe on the following page.)

4 T	Salted Butter-Softened
2 T, 2 t	Erythritol
1/4 t	Vanilla Extract
1/4 t	Salt
1/8 C	Sugar Free Chocolate Chip Cookie Dough Syrup (Such as Torani)
1 C	Almond Flour
2 T, 2 t	Dark Chocolate Chips (Such as Lily's)

In a large bowl, cream together the first five ingredients until combined.

Slowly add in the almond flour, creaming until fully incorporated.

Smash or chop the chocolate chips and fold into the cookie dough.

Cover with plastic wrap and refrigerate until somewhat firm, 15 to 20 minutes.

Shape firm dough into marble-sized balls, and freeze solid.

(Nutrition facts are incorporated into the ice cream nutrition on the following page.)

Cookie Dough
(Makes 2 Quarts = 16 Servings of 1/2 Cup)

2 C	Unsweetened Coconut Milk
2 Cans	Unsweetened Coconut Cream
2 T	Erythritol
1/2 C	Sugar Substitute (Such as Stevia or Splenda)
1/2 t	Salt
1 1/2 T	Vanilla Extract
1 t	Xanthan Gum
2 t	Sugar Substitute (Such as Stevia or Splenda)
1 C	Sugar Free Cookie Dough Syrup (Such as Torani)
1/2 C	Cookie Dough Bits (From recipe on previous page)

*You will need rock salt and a good supply of ice.

In a large saucepan, add first six ingredients. Warm the mixture on medium-low to low heat, dissolving the lumps of coconut cream. Stir occasionally to determine when the lumps are melted.

Once the lumps are dissolved, refrigerate the base ingredients until chilled. (Chill your ice cream canister at this time-if recommended in the ice cream maker's instructions.)

In a tiny bowl, mix together the xanthan gum and sugar substitute and set aside until your base mixture is chilled. When the base mixture is chilled, add the Cookie Dough syrup and pour into a blender. Sprinkle the xanthan/sugar substitute mixture on top and blend for 30 seconds to a minute.

Empty the liquid mixture into your ice cream canister, using a spatula if necessary. Churn, following the ice cream maker's instructions.

Pour into a freezer-safe container, allowing for expansion of ingredients, and stir in the Cookie Dough bits from the recipe on previous page. Eat immediately as soft serve, or chill 2-4 hours.

Nutrition Per Serving (1/2 Cup):
Calories: 140; Fat: 11g: Sat Fat 10g; Protein: <1g; Carbs: 2g, 1g as Erythritol

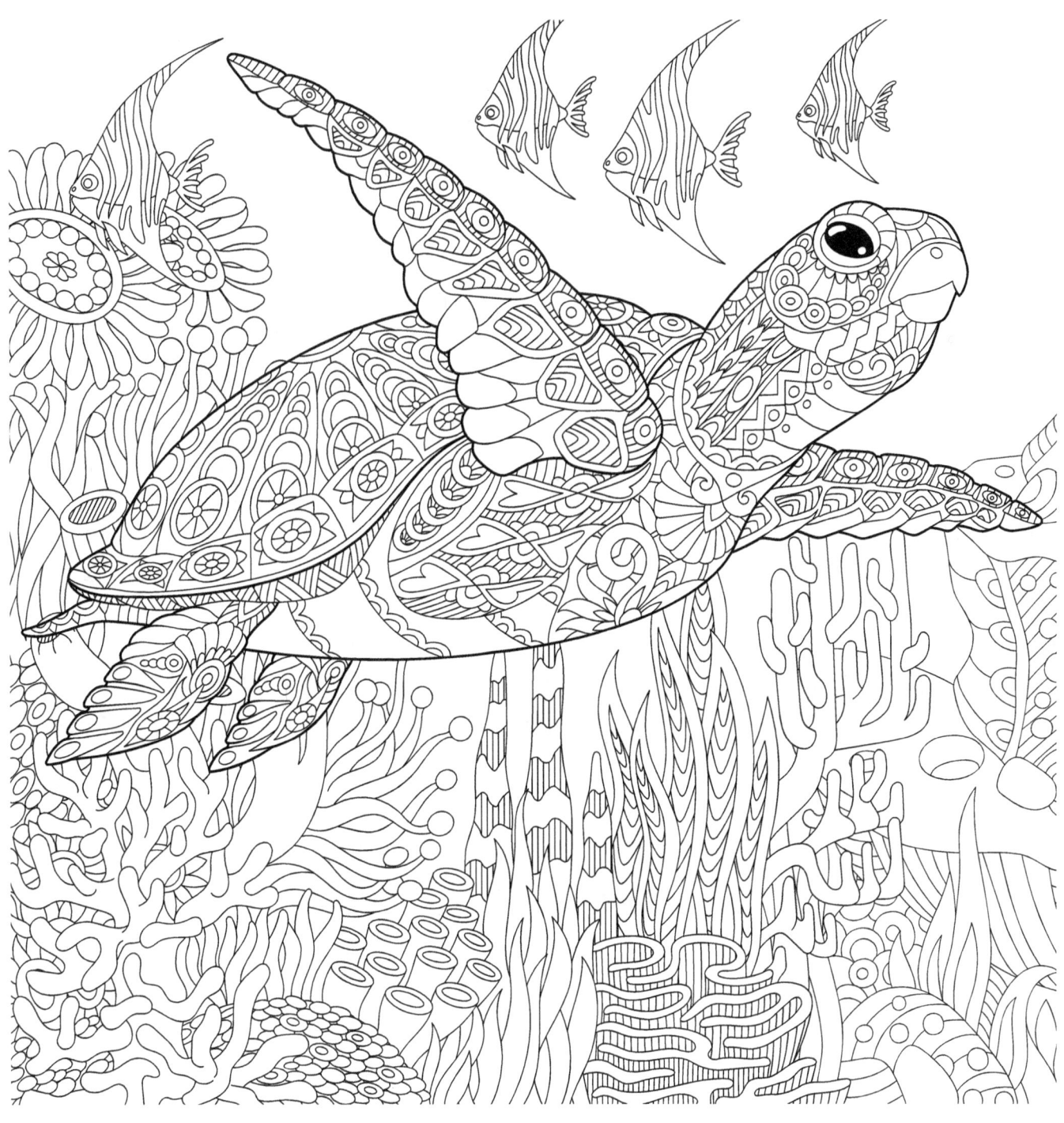

Moose Track Bits

(This makes enough for the 2 Quart Ice Cream recipe on the following page.)

1 C	Creamy Peanut Butter Natural, no sugar added (Such as Smuckers)
1/2 C	Powdered Erythritol
1/2 C	Dark Chocolate Chips (Such as Lily's) Smashed or chopped

Cream together the peanut butter and powdered erythritol.

Add the chocolate chips bits.

Shape into marble-sized balls, and freeze solid.

(Nutrition facts are incorporated into the ice cream nutrition on the following page.)

Moose Tracks
(Makes 2 Quarts = 16 Servings of 1/2 Cup)

2 C	Unsweetened Coconut Milk
2 Cans	Unsweetened Coconut Cream
2 T	Erythritol
1/2 C	Sugar Substitute (Such as Splenda)
1/2 t	Salt
1 1/2 T	Vanilla Extract
1 t	Xanthan Gum
2 t	Sugar Substitute (Such as Stevia or Splenda)
1 C	Sugar Free Vanilla Bean Syrup (Such as Torani)
1/2 C	Moose Track Bits (From recipe on previous page)

*You will need rock salt and a good supply of ice.

In a large saucepan, add the first six ingredients. Warm the mixture on medium-low to low heat, dissolving the lumps of coconut cream.

Once the lumps are dissolved, refrigerate the base ingredients until chilled. (Chill your ice cream canister at this time-if recommended in the ice cream maker's instructions.)

In a tiny bowl, mix together the xanthan gum and sugar substitute and set aside until the base mixture is chilled. When the base mixture is chilled, add the Vanilla Bean syrup and pour into a blender. Sprinkle the xanthan/sugar substitute mixture on top and blend for 30 seconds to a minute. Empty the liquid mixture into your ice cream canister, using a spatula if necessary. Churn, following the ice cream maker's instructions.

Pour into a freezer-safe container, allowing for expansion of ingredients, and stir in the Moose Track bits from the recipe on previous page. Eat immediately as soft serve, or chill 2-4 hours.

Nutrition Per Serving (1/2 Cup):
Calories: 132; Fat: 12g: Sat Fat 11g; Protein: 1g; Carbs: 3g, 1g as Erythritol

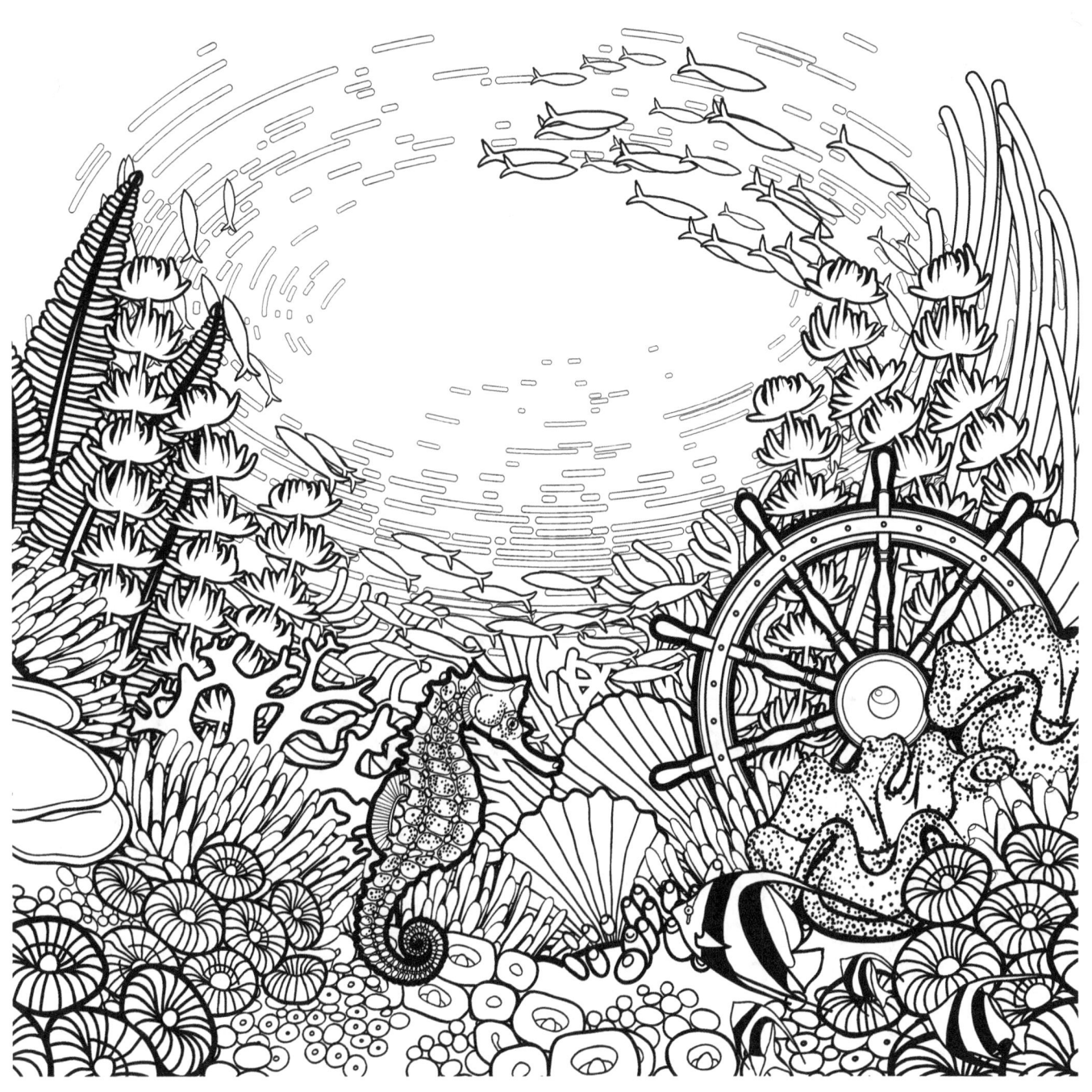

Chocolate Chip Mint
(Makes 2 Quarts = 16 Servings of 1/2 Cup)

2 C	Unsweetened Coconut Milk
2 Cans	Unsweetened Coconut Cream
2 T	Erythritol
1/2 C	Sugar Substitute (Such as Stevia or Splenda)
1/2 t	Salt
1 t	Xanthan Gum
2 t	Sugar Substitute (Such as Stevia or Splenda)
1 C	Sugar Free Chocolate Syrup (Such as Torani)
1/4 C	Chocolate Chip Mint Flavor Fountain (Such as OliveNation)
1/2 C	Dark Chocolate Chips (Such as Lilly's) Chopped or smashed into bits.

*You will need rock salt and a good supply of ice.

In a large saucepan, add first five ingredients. Warm the mixture on medium-low to low heat, dissolving the lumps of coconut cream. As with all previous recipes, this mixture doesn't need to get hot. Dissolve the lumps, stirring occasionally to see if the lumps are melted.

Once the lumps are dissolved, refrigerate the base ingredients until chilled. (Chill your ice cream canister at this time-if recommended in the ice cream maker's instructions.)

In a tiny bowl or ramekin, mix together the xanthan gum and sugar substitute and set aside until the base mixture is chilled. When your base is chilled, add the chocolate syrup and flavor fountain, and pour into a blender. Sprinkle the xanthan/sugar substitute mixture on top and blend for 30 seconds to a minute.

Empty ice cream mixture into your ice cream canister, using a spatula if necessary. Churn, following the ice cream maker's instructions.

Pour into a freezer-safe container, allowing for expansion of ingredients, and stir in the dark chocolate chip bits. Eat immediately as soft serve, or chill 2-4 hours.

Nutrition Per Serving (1/2 Cup):
Calories: 127; Fat: 12g: Sat Fat 11g; Protein: <1g; Carbs: 5g, 3g as Erythritol

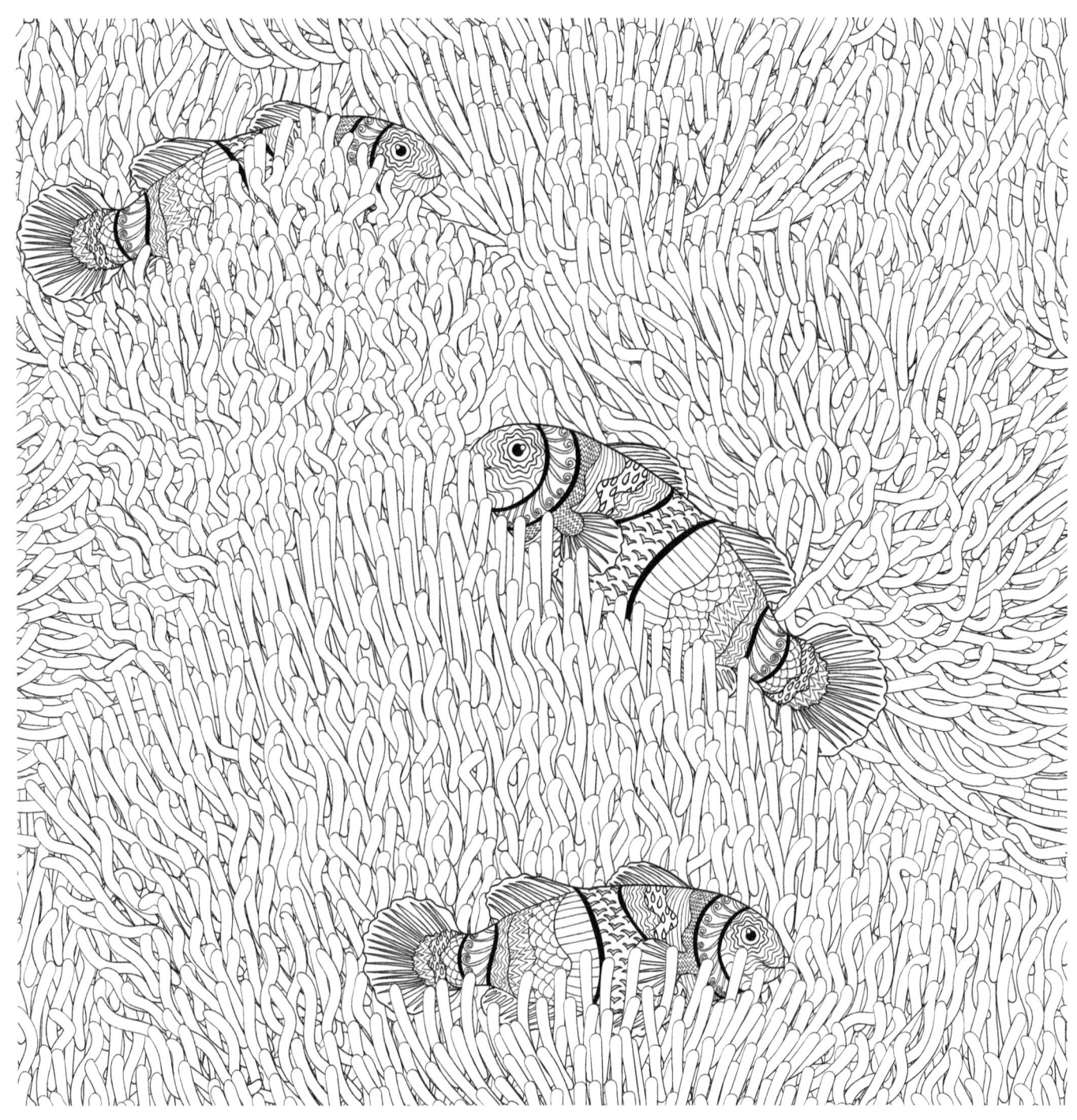

Graham Cracker Bits

(This makes enough for the 2 Quart Ice Cream recipe on the following page.)

1/2 C	Almond Flour
1 T, 1 t	Sugar Substitute (Splenda)
1/2 t	Cinnamon
1/4 t	Baking Powder
Smidge	Salt
2 1/4 t	Liquid Egg (Or 1/4 of a Large Egg)
1/2 T	Butter-Melted
1/2 t	Molasses
1/4 t	Vanilla Extract

Preheat oven to 300°

Mix the first five ingredients in a bowl.

Stir in the last four ingredients until it's a well combined dough.

Spread a piece of parchment paper on the counter and place the dough on top. Pat the dough into a square. Place another piece of parchment on top and roll the dough evenly until it's about 1/8" to 1/4" thick.

Remove the top piece of parchment. Place the dough and under-parchment onto a baking sheet.

Bake 20-30 minutes until the crackers are browning and firming. Remove from oven, turning it off, and let cool 30 minutes.

Return the crackers to the turned-off oven, but still warm oven. If the oven is cooled completely, turn on to 200° or less. Leave in for 30 minutes or so and remove to cool and firm.

Break the firm crackers into tiny rectangles. These will be mixed with ice cream, so make them no bigger than a quarter of a postage stamp. They don't need to be a uniform size.

Freeze the bits solid.

(Nutrition facts are incorporated into the ice cream nutrition on the following page.)

Banana Cream Pie
(Makes 2 Quarts = 16 Servings of 1/2 Cup)

2 C	Unsweetened Coconut Milk
2 Cans	Unsweetened Coconut Cream
2 T	Erythritol
1/2 C	Sugar Substitute (Such as Stevia or Splenda)
1/2 t	Salt
1 t	Xanthan Gum
2 t	Sugar Substitute (Splenda)
1 C	Sugar Free Banana Syrup (Such as Da Vinci)
1/2 C	Graham Cracker Bits (From recipe on previous page)

*You will need rock salt and a good supply of ice.

In a large saucepan, add the first five ingredients. Warm the mixture on medium-low to low heat, dissolving the lumps of coconut cream. This mixture doesn't need to get hot, just melt the lumps.

Once the lumps are dissolved, refrigerate the base ingredients until chilled. (Chill your ice cream canister at this time-if recommended in the ice cream maker's instructions.)

In a tiny bowl, mix together the xanthan gum and sugar substitute. Set aside. When the base ingredients are chilled, add the banana syrup and pour into a blender. Sprinkle the xanthan/sugar substitute mixture on top and blend for 30 seconds to a minute. Empty the liquid ice cream mixture into your ice cream canister, using a spatula if necessary. Churn, following the ice cream maker's instructions.

Pour into a freezer-safe container, allowing for expansion of ingredients, and stir in the Graham Cracker bits from the recipe on previous page. Eat immediately as soft serve, or chill 2-4 hours.

Nutrition Per Serving (1/2 Cup):
Calories: 126; Fat: 12g: Sat Fat 10g; Protein: <1g; Carbs: 2g, 1g as Erythritol

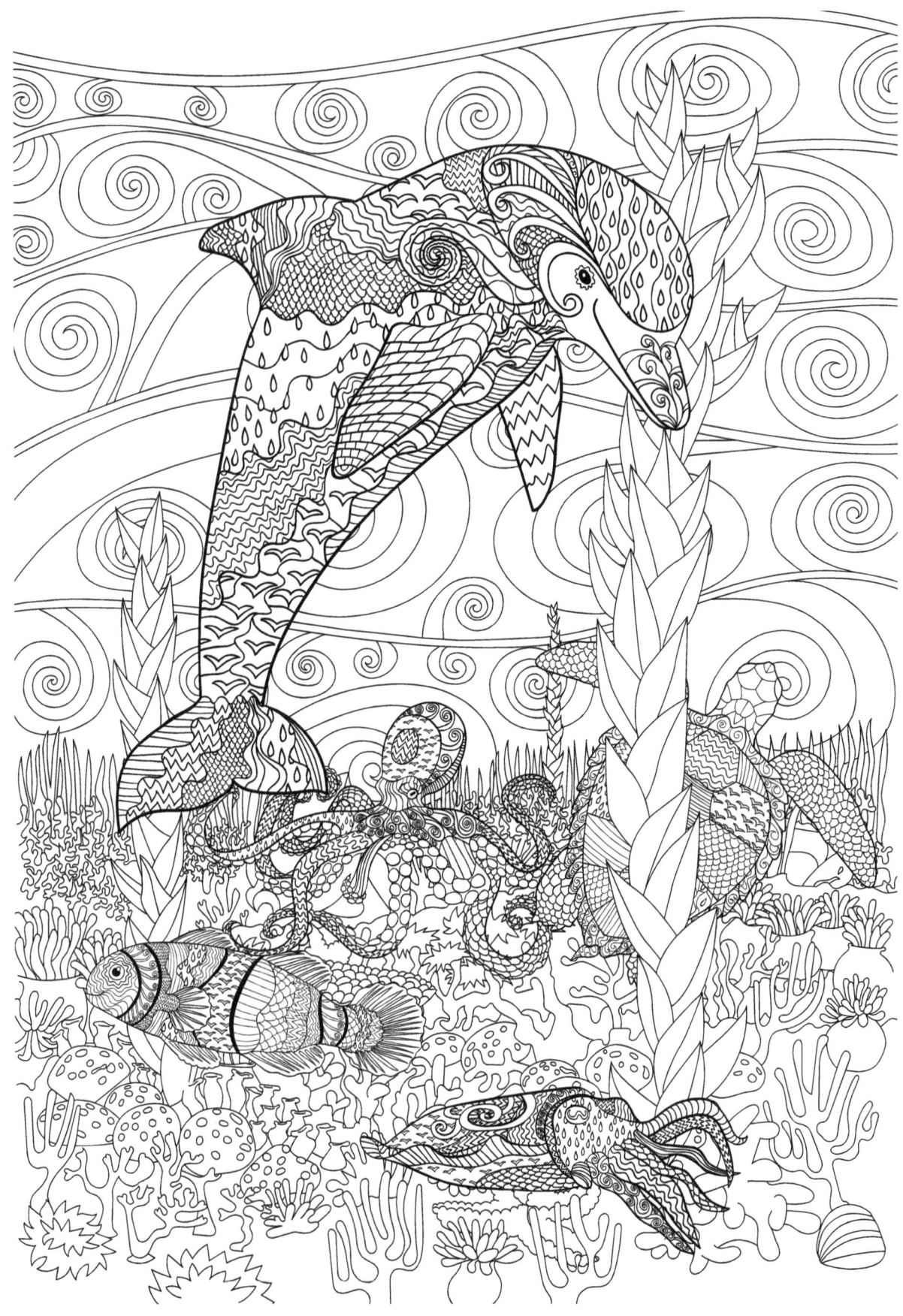

Keto Brown Sugar

(This makes enough for the 2 Quart Ice Cream recipe on the following page.)

1/3 C	Erythritol
1/2 t	Molasses
1/2 t	Liquid Stevia or stevia glycerite

In a small bowl, combine all three ingredients. I find it easiest to get in there with clean hands and mush/sift the ingredients together.

Add this to the base ingredients on the following page.

(Nutrition facts are incorporated into the ice cream nutrition.)

Butter Pecan
(Makes 2 Quarts = 16 Servings of 1/2 Cup)

2 C	Unsweetened Coconut Milk
2 Cans	Unsweetened Coconut Cream
2 T	Erythritol
1/2 C	Sugar Substitute (Such as Stevia or Splenda)
1/2 t	Salt
1 1/2 T	Vanilla Extract
All	Keto Brown Sugar (from recipe on previous page)
1 t	Xanthan Gum
2 t	Sugar Substitute (Such as Stevia or Splenda)
3/4 C	Chopped Pecans
2 T	Salted Butter

*You will need rock salt and a good supply of ice.

In a large saucepan, combine the first seven ingredients. Warm the mixture on medium-low to low heat, dissolving the lumps of coconut cream. Once the lumps are dissolved, refrigerate the base ingredients until chilled. (Chill your ice cream canister.)

In a tiny bowl, mix together the xanthan gum and sugar substitute. Set aside. When the base mixture is chilled, start toasting your chopped pecans: Place the butter in a small frying pan, on medium/low-low heat. Add the pecans, stirring occasionally with a spatula, 5-7 minutes until the pecans are toasted and the butter is bubbly-thick and brown.

While the pecans are toasting, pour your chilled base mixture into a blender. Sprinkle xanthan/sugar substitute mixture on top and blend for 30 seconds to a minute. Empty the liquid ice cream mixture into your ice cream canister, using a spatula if necessary and scrape the toasted pecans on top of mixture, making sure to get every bit of browned butter. Churn, following the ice cream maker's instructions.

Eat immediately as soft serve, or pour into a freezer-safe container, allowing for expansion of ingredients, and chill 2-4 hours.

Nutrition Per Serving (1/2 Cup):
Calories: 162; Fat: 16g: Sat Fat 10g; Protein: 2g; Carbs: 5g, 4g as Erythritol

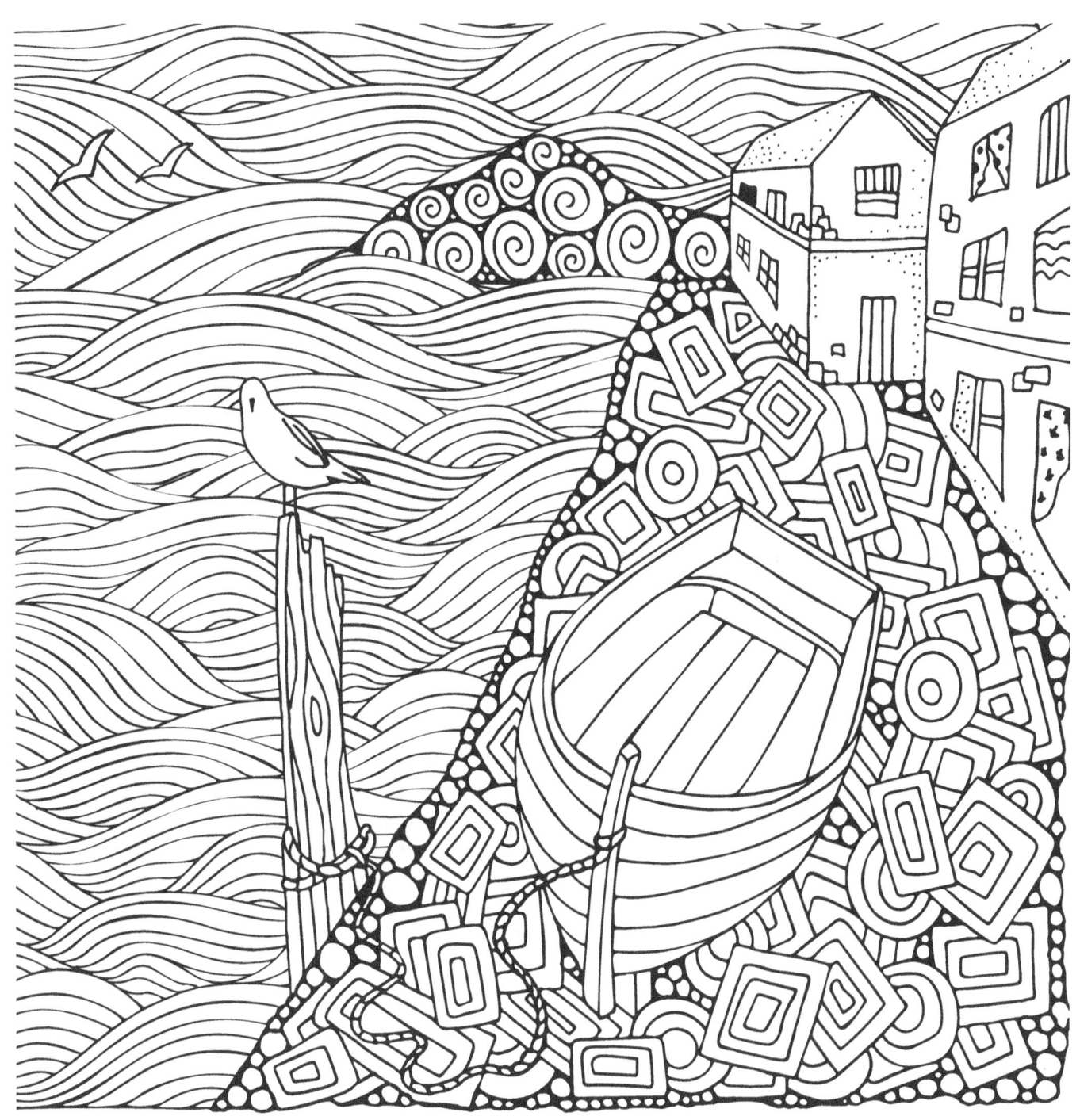

Caramel Pecan
(Makes 2 Quarts = 16 Servings of 1/2 Cup)

2 C	Unsweetened Coconut Milk
2 Cans	Unsweetened Coconut Cream
2 T	Erythritol
1/2 C	Sugar Substitute (Such as Stevia or Splenda)
1/2 t	Salt
1 t	Xanthan Gum
2 t	Sugar Substitute (Such as Stevia or Splenda)
1 C	Sugar Free Caramel Syrup (Such as Torani)
1/2 C	Chopped Pecans

*You will need rock salt and a good supply of ice.

In a large saucepan, add the first five ingredients. Warm the mixture on medium-low to low heat, dissolving the lumps of coconut cream. Dissolve the lumps, while stirring occasionally to see if they're melted.

Once the lumps are dissolved, refrigerate the base ingredients until chilled. (Chill your ice cream canister at this time-if recommended in the ice cream maker's instructions.)

In a tiny bowl, mix together the xanthan gum and sugar substitute and set aside. When your base mixture is chilled, add the caramel syrup and pour into a blender. Sprinkle the xanthan/sugar substitute mixture on top and blend for 30 seconds to a minute.

Empty the liquid ice cream mixture into your ice cream canister, using a spatula if necessary. Churn, following the ice cream maker's instructions.

Pour into a freezer-safe container, allowing for expansion of ingredients, and stir in the chopped pecans. Eat immediately as soft serve, or chill 2-4 hours.

Nutrition Per Serving (1/2 Cup):
Calories: 149; Fat: 15g: Sat Fat 10g; Protein: <1g; Carbs: 2g, 1g as Erythritol

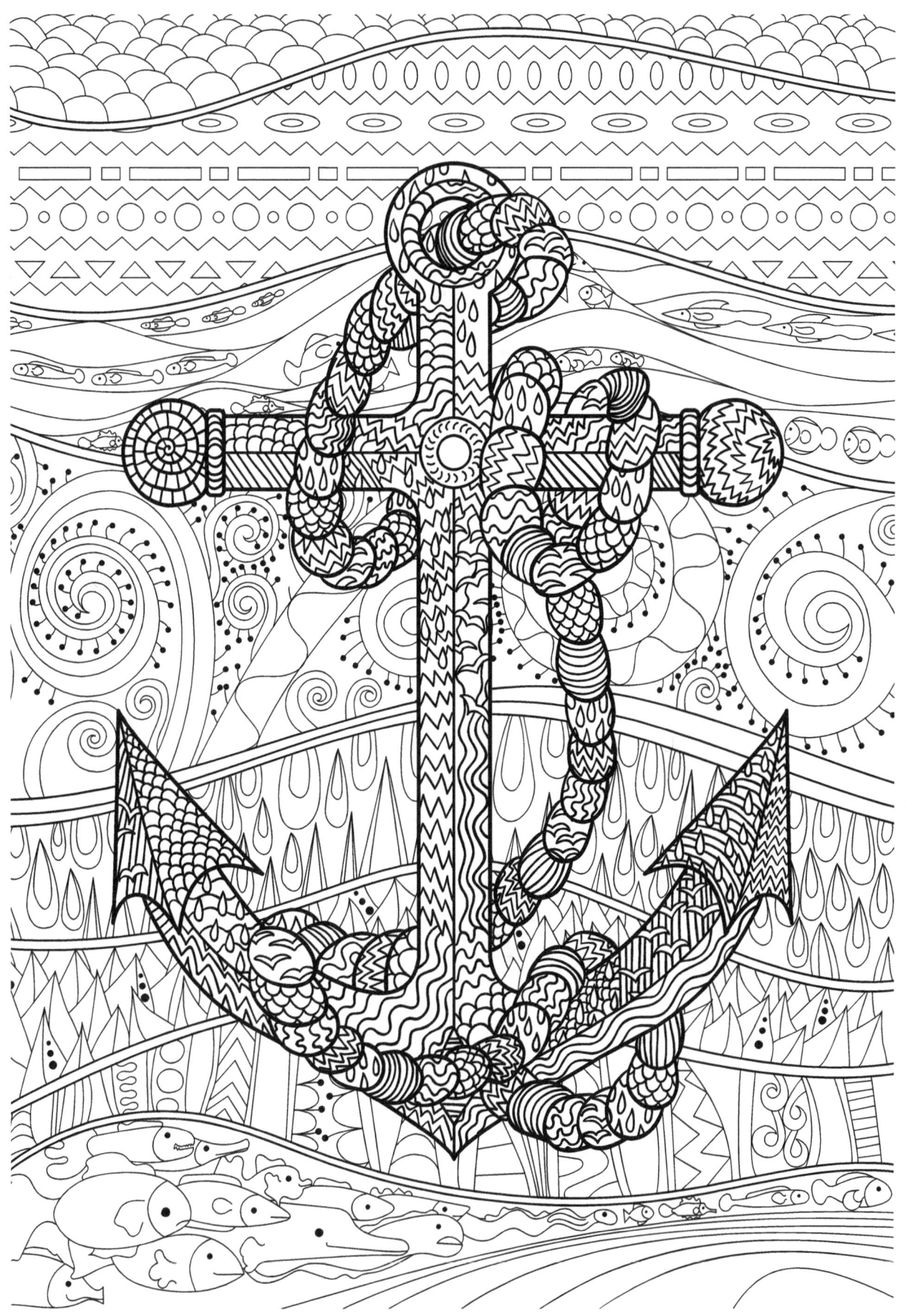

Cherry Nut
(Makes 2 Quarts = 16 Servings of 1/2 Cup)

2 C	Unsweetened Coconut Milk
2 Cans	Unsweetened Coconut Cream
2 T	Erythritol
1/2 C	Sugar Substitute (Such as Stevia or Splenda)
1/2 t	Salt
1 1/2 T	Pure Cherry Extract
1 t	Xanthan Gum
2 t	Sugar Substitute (Such as Stevia or Splenda)
1 C	Sugar Free Cherry Syrup (I used "Time For Treats")
1/2 C	Chopped Walnuts

*You will need rock salt and a good supply of ice.

In a large saucepan, add the first six ingredients. Warm the mixture on medium-low to low heat, dissolving the lumps of coconut cream. You know the drill; this mixture doesn't need to get hot. Stir occasionally until the lumps are melted.

Once the lumps are dissolved, refrigerate the base ingredients until chilled. (Chill your ice cream canister at this time-if recommended in the ice cream maker's instructions.)

In a tiny bowl, mix together the xanthan gum and sugar substitute and set aside. When the base mixture is chilled, add the cherry syrup and pour into a blender. Sprinkle the xanthan/sugar substitute mixture on top and blend for 30 seconds to a minute.

Empty ice cream mixture into your ice cream canister, using a spatula if necessary. Churn, following the ice cream maker's instructions.

Pour into a freezer-safe container, allowing for expansion of ingredients, and stir in the chopped walnuts. Eat immediately as soft serve, or chill 2-4 hours.

Nutrition Per Serving (1/2 Cup):
Calories: 147; Fat: 14g: Sat Fat 10g; Protein: 1g; Carbs: 2g, 1g as Erythritol

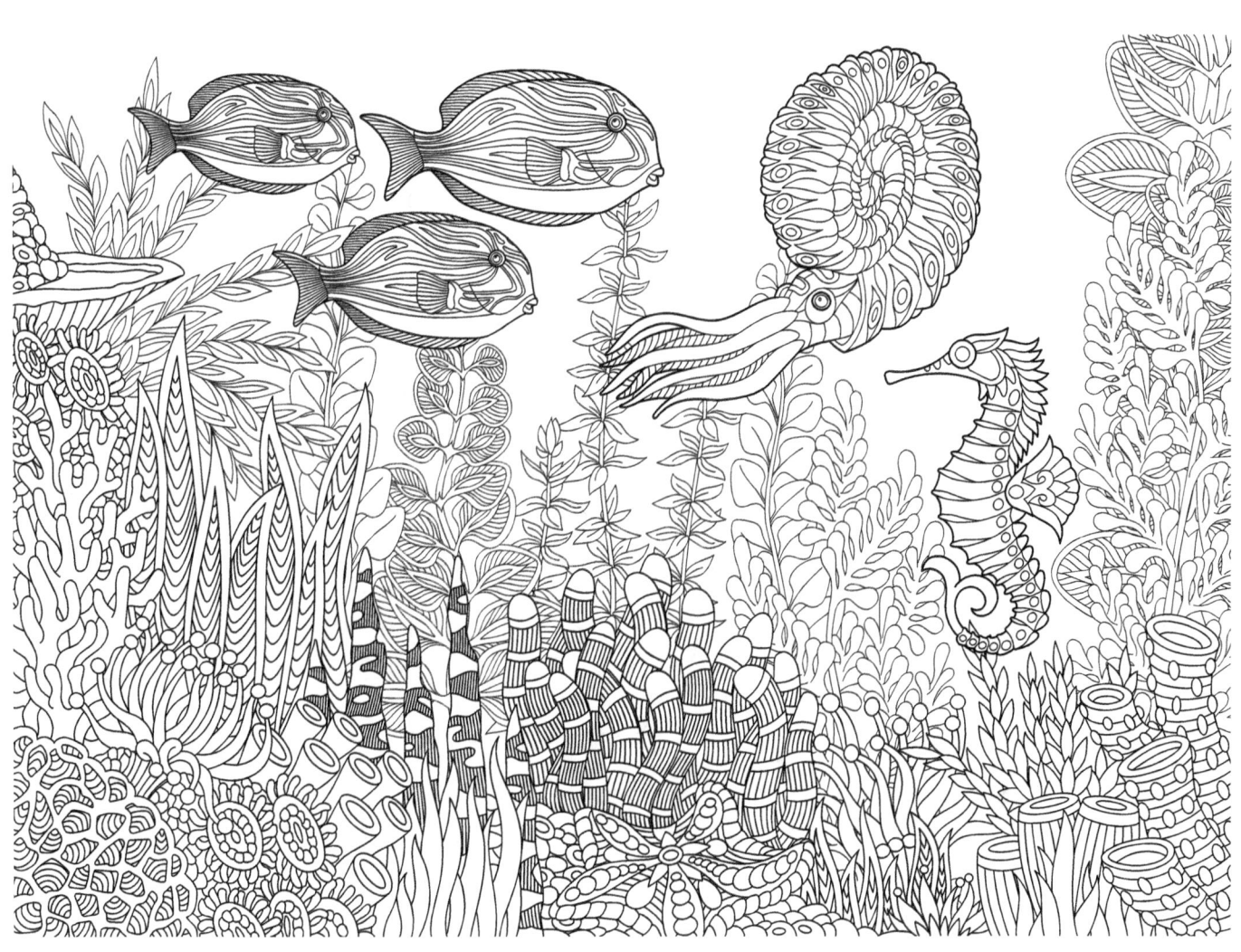

Recipe Notes

Most of the time, when I'm making ice cream I make a variety of flavors, but I don't necessarily want to make 2 quarts of each. I'd be churning for hours and I'd have no place to put them all. So I've developed a versatile base, making it easy to whip up a full batch of ice cream and separate it into halves or quarters, flavoring it according to craving. On the next page, I've set out the base ingredients, and their conversion amounts.

With these conversions, you can make whatever amounts of each flavor you prefer. Or, experiment with smaller batches yourself, coming up with your own flavor profiles.

Simply make as many of the full recipes as you'd like at one time, and divide them however you please before adding any flavoring. And don't worry if you decide to wave the white flag and surrender for the day. I have, on occasion, overestimated my batch-churning stamina. Happily, this base can keep in the refrigerator, in a sealed container, for a day or two.

So, here are the basics for multi-batches, as stated in the preceding recipes:

In a large saucepan, add the full recipe amount or half recipe amount of the first five ingredients. (Follow the conversion amounts on the facing page.)

(*Some of the recipes have extract, which is a sixth ingredient. I recommend heating extracts with the base if you're making full recipes of these. However, if you're going to make partial batches of these, it's okay to add the extract after the refrigeration process, before putting in the blender.)

Warm the mixture on medium-low to low heat, dissolving the lumps of coconut cream as stated in all of the recipes.

Once the lumps are dissolved, refrigerate until chilled while chilling your ice cream canister-if recommended in the ice cream maker's instructions.

When the base mixture is chilled, use the conversions on the facing page to divide a full recipe to your liking and follow the rest of each recipe's instructions.

*One note regarding Xanthan. You may find you like your ice cream icier or creamier. Adjust Xanthan/Splenda mixture accordingly. Less Xanthan will make it icier, more makes it creamier.

*And remember, for multiple recipes, you'll need rock salt and lots of ice.

Ice Cream Base & Conversion Amounts

Base Ingredient Recipe:

Full Recipe (5 1/2 C of liquid)		1/2 Recipe (2 3/4 C of liquid)
2 C	Coconut Milk	1 C
2 Cans	Coconut Cream	1 Can
2T	Erythritol	1 T
1/2 C	Splenda	1/4 C
1/2 t	Salt	1/4 t

Warm on Med-Low until sugars and cream dissolve. Refrigerate.

Before blending, measure out the amount of base you want. As shown below, a full recipe of 2 frozen quarts of ice cream equals 5 1/2 cups of liquid. A half recipe, or 1 quart of ice cream, equals 2 3/4 cups of liquid. And a quarter recipe, or a half a quart of frozen ice cream, equals 1 1/3 cups of liquid).

Then add corresponding flavors, xanthan gum thickener/Splenda, and bits according to the chart.

Base Ingredient liquid Measurements:

Full Recipe = 5 1/2 C	1/2 Recipe = 2 3/4 C	1/4 Recipe = 1 1/3 C

Flavorings, thickener amounts, and other added bits:

1 C	Syrup	1/2 C	1/4 C
1 1/2 T	*Extract	2 1/4 t	1 1/8 t
1/4 C	*Flavor Fountain	1/8 C	1 T
1/4 C	*Cocoa Powder	1/8 C	1 T
1 t	Xanthan Gum	1/2 t	1/4 t
2 t	Splenda	1 t	1/2 t
1/2 C	**Bits	1/4 C	1/8 C

(*Some recipes have extract, powder, or flavor fountain flavorings in addition to the sugar free syrup)
(**Bits are chocolate chips, nuts, moose track bits, cookie dough bits, graham cracker bits, etc...)

Thank you for purchasing my book!
(If you enjoyed it, please consider leaving a review.)

Keep in touch and be in the loop for upcoming coloring cookbooks:

www.suzysable.com
https://www.instagram.com/authorsuzysable/

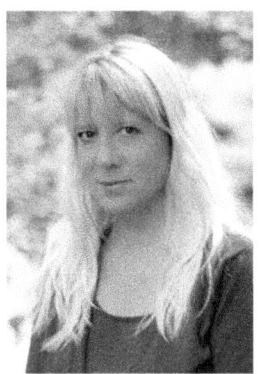

Suzy Sable lives in the Midwest, and has been pinch-and-dash cooking since she was a teen. Nestled north of Minneapolis, MN, USA, she hunkers down in the freezing winters, passing the time in her cozy, warm kitchen.

She's always loved to adapt recipes, tasting and tinkering until she gets them juu-ust right! She admits that all that tasting and tinkering widened her waistline...until she started eating keto.

So, for her it was a pleasure and a challenge to work with the unfamiliar keto ingredients, whipping up delights to please the palate as well as the body.

Get in touch with Suzy on the Contact page of her website:

www.suzysable.com